Diet only half the time . . . but get twice the results!

"A variation [on periodic fasting] that also may lead to weight loss is restricting calories on alternate days. In a small study published in March, researchers followed a group of ten people with a body mass index above 30 who were fed just 20 percent of their normal calorie intake on alternate days. On the other days they could eat what they wanted. After eight weeks, they'd lost an average of 8 percent of their body weight. These people were also asthma patients, and their symptoms also improved significantly after two weeks on the regimen."

—*US News & World Report*

Discover the breakthrough technique that allows you to activate your "skinny gene" and enjoy these remarkable and measurable benefits:

- Lose fat easily and quickly without deprivation, discomfort, or stress.

- Improve fat metabolism.

- Avoid regaining lost fat.

- Slow the aging process.

- Optimize nutrition.

- Reduce by as much as 90 percent the primary cause of inflammatory disease.

The

Alternate-Day

Diet

THE ORIGINAL UP-DAY, DOWN-DAY EATING
PLAN TO TURN ON YOUR "SKINNY GENE,"
SHED THE POUNDS, AND LIVE A LONGER
AND HEALTHIER LIFE

Updated and Revised

James B. Johnson, MD

with Donald R. Laub Sr., MD

A PERIGEE BOOK

A PERIGEE BOOK
Published by the Penguin Group
Penguin Group (USA) LLC
375 Hudson Street, New York, New York 10014

USA • Canada • UK • Ireland • Australia • New Zealand • India • South Africa • China

penguin.com

A Penguin Random House Company

Revised Perigee trade paperback ISBN: 978-0-399-16703-4

The Library of Congress has cataloged the Perigee hardcover edition as follows:

Johnson, James B., MD.
The alternate-day diet : turn on your skinny gene, shed the pounds,
and live a longer and healthier life /
James B. Johnson with Donald R. Laub.
p.   cm.
ISBN 978-0-399-15493-5
1. Reducing diets.   2. Nutrition—Genetic aspects.   3. Low-calorie diet.
I. Laub, Donald R.   II. Title
RM222.2.J554   2008   2008005400
613.2′5—dc22

PUBLISHING HISTORY
G. P. Putnam's Sons hardcover edition / April 2008
Perigee trade paperback edition / April 2009
Revised Perigee trade paperback edition / January 2014

PRINTED IN THE UNITED STATES OF AMERICA

10 9 8 7 6 5 4 3 2 1

Interior illustrations by Bayard Colyear

Most Perigee books are available at special quantity discounts for bulk purchases for sales
promotions, premiums, fund-raising, or educational use. Special books, or book excerpts, can also
be created to fit specific needs. For details, write: Special.Markets@us.penguingroup.com.

To Dana and Judy, for suffering along with us

Contents

Part One: How I Arrived at This Plan and Why I Know It Works

Part Two: The Alternate-Day Diet Program

Why This Diet?

I have struggled most of my life to maintain a healthy weight. As a plastic surgeon performing liposuction, I have counseled thousands of patients about their weight. Until a few years ago, however, my advice appeared to be inadequate, because very few of my patients lost weight and kept it off. Then, in 2003, I had a weight-loss epiphany. I read about an experiment done on some fat mice at the National Institutes of Health that changed my life.

If you're having trouble controlling your own weight, you may be at least somewhat relieved to know that there is significant scientific research showing that fewer than 10 percent of Americans can eat freely, without restraint, and not gain weight. Sixty-five percent of us either don't restrain or try unsuccessfully, and are, therefore, overweight or obese. That leaves approximately 25 percent of the population who, presumably, restrain successfully and avoid gaining weight.

Since you're reading this, I assume you belong to that 65 percent who fall prey to the fatal attraction of food. If so, you should know that I am just like you. I love to eat food that tastes good and

I used to be hungry—or at least thought I was hungry—virtually all the time.

That's really not so surprising if you consider that when our hunter-gatherer ancestors roamed the earth they truly never knew where their next meal was coming from, and so, whenever there was food available, they ate it. Those who hunted or gathered and ate the most survived, and gradually, over time, that eat-whatever-you-can-whenever-you-can survival instinct was programmed into our DNA. It became part of our genetic code. Now, of course, there's no shortage of food. Good, tasty, inexpensive food is available to all of us in abundance all the time. And our DNA is telling us to eat it.

Going on a diet is, therefore, going against everything our genes are telling us we need to do to survive. In her book *Rethinking Thin*, Gina Kolata, a science writer for the *New York Times*, looks at the plethora of evidence indicating that some people are more genetically predisposed than others to be overweight and concludes that those who are genetically destined to be fat may be incapable of losing a significant amount of weight and keeping it off. *But* she also writes that "the genes that make people fat need an environment in which food is cheap and plentiful," and that is exactly the environment in which we live today. Moreover, if genetics were solely responsible for the epidemic of overweight people in America, it would mean that 65 percent of the population had been born with some kind of rogue fat gene, and there doesn't appear to be any evidence that's true.

When I was a child, my parents had a cabin in northern Michigan where we went for weekends. On the drive home one Sunday we stopped at a place called McDonald's. The hamburgers were tiny, but the french fries and shakes were (and still are) the best I'd ever had. From that day on, stopping at McDonald's became the highlight of my entire weekend. In those days, however, McDonald's locations were few and far between; today it seems there's one on almost every corner—along with Wendy's, Burger King, Dunkin' Donuts, Cinnabon, and thousands of other inexpensive, really tasty, fattening fast-food outlets. Given the combination of our hardwired disposition to eat and a landscape literally littered with tasty food, it's no wonder that, according to a study published in the *Journal of the American Medical Association*, the obesity rate for adults doubled between 1980 and 2002.

Despite these obstacles, however, the majority of us continue to try to lose weight because we don't like the way we look or feel. We want to fit into attractive clothes, we want to have more energy, and we want to live longer. And whatever nature or nurture, biology or environment tells us about our chances for success, we seem to keep on trying. A 2007 article in the Health section of the *Washington Post* reported that one in three American adults are trying to lose weight at any given time.

Like you, I've been on any number of diets, all of which worked so long as I stuck with them. But inevitably, at some point, "diet fatigue" set in and the predisposition to eat everything that came my way won out. I fell off the wagon, so to speak, and gained back whatever weight I'd lost. I'm sure you've been there too.

Where I may be different from you, however, is that, as a medical doctor, I have access to and am familiar with much of the scientific research showing how and why nutrition affects longevity and health. In fact, as you will see, I've conducted some of that research myself.

For years I was familiar with the work being done primarily by Roy Walford and his colleagues at UCLA, which showed that severely restricting our caloric intake would substantially prolong our life and health. Even knowing that, however, I was conscious enough of my own limitations to understand that I couldn't or wouldn't subject myself to such radical food deprivation for any length of time.

The breakthrough for me came when I read about a study done by Mark Mattson and his colleagues at the National Institute on Aging. What these researchers discovered was that mice who were fed only on alternate days and who were allowed to eat as much as they wanted on the days they were fed, experienced as great or greater health benefits as a control group of mice who were fed a restricted diet on a daily basis.

I knew I wouldn't be able to fast on alternate days, but I thought I might be able to restrict my calorie intake enough every other day to reap the same health benefits as those mice. I decided to become my own guinea pig (or lab mouse) and began to restrict my calories to 20 percent of what I normally ate on alternate days. On nonrestrictive days I ate whatever and as much as I wanted.

A couple of weeks into my self-designed program I realized that I was losing weight. I lost 35 pounds in the first 11 weeks and have kept that weight off since 2003. I did not feel deprived or frustrated, as I had on other diets I'd tried, and many of the hundreds of patients I have put on this plan since that time have experienced similar results.

As you read on, you'll learn how and why the Alternate-Day Diet works. You'll hear about how you can activate a magic gene called SIRT1 that not only prevents and repairs the damage done to our cells by free radicals but also inhibits our ability to store fat. Once you understand the scientific evidence supporting the efficacy of alternate-day calorie restriction, I believe, you'll have all the trust and motivation you need to begin losing weight and improving your own health and longevity—for the rest of your life.

How does the Alternate-Day Diet work? It's simple. In fact, the goal of the "down day" (when you eat less) is to simplify your food choices so that you won't have to think too much about what you're eating, you'll be less inclined to cheat, and you'll soon learn to differentiate between true hunger and the desire for a gratifying taste sensation or the need to quench emotional hunger. The "up days" are up to you. You'll be eating what you normally eat, without restriction, as long as you keep calories low on the down days.

You may be thinking that this will never work because you'll be so starving after your down days that you'll binge on your up days and all your effort will be for naught. Happily, however, that simply isn't true. Although we're not yet sure why, people—including me—who go on the diet report that, much to their surprise, they are no hungrier and eat no more on their unrestricted days than they would if they weren't dieting at all.

The proof of the pudding is, as they say, in the eating. But before you turn to the diet itself, I strongly recommend that you read about the underlying science, because doing that will, as I've said, convince you (as it convinced me) of its validity and, therefore, increase your motivation to stick with it long enough to see the benefits for yourself.

Back to the Future: Validating the Alternate-Day Diet

Intermittent fasting, in some form, has been a part of religious observance since ancient times. The ancient Greek Oracle at Delphi is said to have undergone purification rites, including fasting, before delivering her prophesies. Even today, Christians, Jews, and Muslims include some form of fasting or constrained consumption in their religious observances. During the month of Ramadan, Muslims fast from dawn to sunset, eating only one meal before dawn and another to break the fast at sunset. Most Christian religions observe some form of fasting or abstinence—such as abstaining from animal products or "giving up" a favorite food during the forty days of Lent. And Jews fast from sundown on the eve of Yom Kippur, the holiest day in the Jewish calendar, until the following sundown.

What is important to note about these various observances is that they create physical deprivation that is intended and believed to increase spiritual observance. They are not meant to be easy or "fun" holidays, and the only reason that people are willing and able to comply with their restrictions is that they last only for a limited period of time.

Limiting deprivation while increasing health and longevity is also the basis for the development of what I call the "up-day, down-day diet," which became the basis for this book. I was initially inspired to develop the diet by reading about a mouse study done in 2003 by Mark Mattson and his colleagues at the National Institute on Aging. Mattson discovered that when mice specifically bred to gorge themselves were fed every other day, they ate enough on the alternate feeding days to compensate for the fasting days and, therefore, to maintain their weight. Despite their lack of weight loss, however, their markers for longevity and resistance to brain injury were more significantly improved than those of a second group of the same breed of mice who were fed freely every day or than the markers of a third group who were given only 60 percent of their normal calorie intake on a daily basis. Those in the last group not surprisingly lost weight, and while the logical supposition would be that the thin mice would also the healthiest, that was not what Mattson found.

I was stunned by the results of this study. If the same applied to humans, it would mean that by following an alternate-day calorie reduction we would be healthier even if we were fat, thereby defying the conventional wisdom that becoming thin is the only road to optimal health.

The only problem was that I knew I wouldn't be able to eat *nothing* every other day for any significant length of time. I decided that the minimum number of calories I could tolerate on the restricted days would be 20 percent of my normal calorie requirement, and I believed for a variety of reasons that this level would be low enough to trigger the health benefits seen by Mattson in his mice. On the normal eating days I would follow my regular diet, which was not always the healthiest, and I wouldn't restrict myself in any way except that I wouldn't overeat.

Within two weeks of putting myself on this diet, I had lost a significant amount of weight and improved my triglyceride and fasting glucose levels. I also had relief from chronic sinusitis and improvement in my arthritis symptoms. It appeared that the diet was working as I had expected it would! I began to proclaim these remarkable effects to my friends, family, and patients, and I encouraged them to try it.

At the same time, I was told by a friend that Eric Ravussin, a well-known metabolic researcher at the Pennington Biomedical Research Center in Baton Rouge, was also interested in the concept of alternate-day restriction, so I called him and described my 20 percent/100 percent diet. He responded that he believed he could go all day without eating anything and told me that he and his colleagues were in the process of setting up a three-week study during which a group of staff members at Pennington would eat nothing every other day.

Ravussin and I met a few weeks later, in September of 2003, at which time I told him of my own experience with the 20 percent/100 percent plan, as well as the results seen by the two hundred or so people to whom I had by then introduced the idea. At the time I was also developing a protocol to study the health effects as well as the weight-loss benefits of my plan specifically in a group of asthma patients. Dr. Ravussin and I shared our opinions and then independently returned to the pursuit of our separate studies.

We didn't correspond again until the following fall, at which point I wrote to tell him that the results of our Asthma Study (which you'll be reading more about in Chapter 4) had been extremely positive in terms of both weight loss and improvement of the participants' asthma symptoms. In fact, no other study before or since has shown such significant improvement from any treatment modality including medications. The cherry on the cake, so to speak, was that they also reported that their mood and energy levels increased throughout the study period and their hunger levels were no worse on the restricted day than on the day they ate freely.

Ravussin responded that he and his colleagues had also completed their study, which had been accepted for publication in the *American Journal of Clinical Nutrition*. At that time, he sent me a copy of the manuscript and wrote in an email on September 10, 2004:

> As you can see from the manuscript we obtained a significant weight loss over a short time period (3 weeks), but unlike in your experience I think that the volunteers of this study did not experience a decrease in hunger over time. I guess maybe the 20% that you allow is providing enough volume to satisfy the people.

In his paper, which was published in January of 2005, Ravussin stated that the objective of the study "was to determine whether alternate-day fasting is a feasible method of dietary restriction in non-obese humans and whether it improves known biomarkers of longevity." He went on to say that the participants did lose weight and that they showed improvement in biomarkers of health. But the article also states that, "hunger on fasting days did not decrease, perhaps indicating the unlikelihood of continuing this diet for extended periods of time. *Adding one small meal on a fasting day may make this approach to dietary restriction more acceptable.*" (Emphasis added.)

In November of 2004, my coauthor, Dr. Donald Laub, and I presented the preliminary results of our study at a national meeting of the Calorie Restriction Society. Dr. Mark Mattson, who was also at the meeting, suggested that his laboratory perform assays not available anywhere except at a research center, on the frozen samples we had collected, and subsequently he collaborated with us on the first published article about the 20 percent/100 percent diet, which appeared in the peer-reviewed journal *Free Radical Biology and Medicine*.

Up to that time, the only study of alternate-day calorie restriction with good nutrition and without total fasting with human beings as its subjects had been conducted in Spain in 1956 by Dr. Eduardo Arias Vallejo. The participants were a group of healthy men and women over the age of sixty-five who were living in an old-age home in Madrid. Vallejo's work had always been considered by later authors to consist of an overall calorie restriction of 35 percent, meaning that the amount the participants ate on their "normal" eating days did not fully compensate for those they lacked on the restricted days. However, as you'll read in Chapter 3, when my colleagues and I revisited the data, we were able to show that (not unlike Mattson's fat mice) Vallejo's participants were eating *more than normal* on the days when they were allowed to eat freely. On restricted days, they were consuming roughly 50 percent of their normal calories, and on the unrestricted days they were eating about 150 percent. And yet, also like Mattson's mice, their diet reduced their risk of serious illness and death by about one-half as compared to those in the control group. This validated my hypothesis that eating more calories than required on one day and fewer than required the next day in a repeating pattern over a period of time provides very significant health benefits even without weight loss.

In fact, at the time I was working on the first edition of this book, the wide range of health benefits to be gained from alternate-day dieting were not widely recognized by the general public even though they were becoming increasingly clear within the scientific community. For example, at about the same time Ravussin and I were completing our studies, Marc Hellerstein, an endocrinologist and researcher at the University of California at Berkeley, and his colleagues were finding that alternate-day calorie restriction could likely reduce the risk for cancer in mice. Donald Laub and I visited Dr. Hellerstein, who had already heard about our 20 percent/100 percent protocol from Eric Ravussin, and discussed our own ongoing findings.

In terms of studying the value for humans of alternate-day restriction without total fasting, I was something of a trailblazer. In August of 2003, I filed a provisional patent for my diet in order to establish a priority date for describing the 20 percent/100 percent pattern, the expected benefits, and the various permutations we have developed since that time. At that point, there had been no publications describing this pattern and virtually all the studies of intermittent fasting, with the exception of Ravussin's, were being done on rodents, for at least a couple of good reasons. First of all, it's much more difficult to get approval for a human study than it is for an animal study, and second, unless the humans are in a closely controlled environment, it's hard to monitor their degree of compliance with the program. A mouse in a cage can eat only what and when you feed it; a human surrounded by supermarkets, restaurants, and street vendors has food available on a daily basis virtually around the clock.

Basically, to develop this diet, I was extrapolating from animal studies and using my understanding of human nature to determine what I thought would be a degree of restriction people would be willing to tolerate that would still provide them with the many health benefits proven in animals. What I arrived at is the diet in this book.

The first two weeks of the Alternate-Day Diet are the most restrictive, allowing only 20 percent of normal calorie intake in the form of a meal replacement shake on alternate days. At that level you will jump-start the health-promoting metabolic changes of the program and also lose significant weight, as did the participants in my Asthma Study. After that, you can start to eat "real food" on the restricted days and can increase your intake to as much as 50 percent of normal caloric needs. The reasons for this are twofold: I believe that almost everyone will find it tolerable, and it has been well established that this level of restriction will both provide the health benefits of alternate-day fasting and also allow for weight maintenance. It is the level that I have maintained for myself.

Of course, if your goal after two weeks is still to lose more weight, the fewer calories you eat on your restricting day, the more weight you're likely to lose—if for no other reason than that you'll be less likely to unthinkingly compensate or even overcompensate for the calorie deficit on the days you eat freely.

Ten years ago, I had to make assumptions and test their validity by applying them in the real world. Since the initial publication of *The Alternate-Day Diet* in 2008, however, other researchers have been validating and duplicating my findings. To date, there has been nothing to alter or invalidate any of the initial assumptions I made all those years ago, nor has there been any significant addition to the underlying science.

What has changed is that the public has now become very aware of the irrefutable benefits of intermittent calorie restriction, and various media have trumpeted the virtues of one version or another of the Alternate-Day Diet as if it were just born yesterday—not unlike the working actor who, after years in the trenches, is suddenly declared an overnight success. One version, for example, suggests restricting for two days and eating normally five days a week. While other forms of intermittent calorie restriction undoubtedly do have benefits, there is no doubt that the pattern I initially conceived remains the most effective.

In terms of validation, one recent study is particularly significant. David Sinclair and his colleagues at Harvard Medical School have now proved beyond any doubt Sinclair's earlier assertion that resveratrol, a compound found in grapes and red wine, improves health and slows the aging process by activating a gene called SIRT1, which is also activated by alternate-day calorie restriction. In Chapter 5, you'll be reading about the mechanism through which SIRT1 is activated and about Sinclair's initial research. For the last several years that research has been criticized and repudiated in studies done by drug companies and in other laboratories. Dr. Sinclair has persisted, however, and has now demonstrated beyond question that not only does the activation of SIRT1 set in motion the amazing effects of alternate-day calorie restriction but also that resveratrol can produce the same results. In the history of human scientific research, there has been no other natural mechanism whose discovery is remotely comparable to the potential benefits of activating SIRT1.

Sinclair is now working on developing a synthetic form of resveratrol. If and when that happens, we may have a way to both prolong health and cure obesity simply by taking a pill. That day is still far in the future, however, and in the meantime the most effective and tolerable way for us food-loving humans to stay young and healthy is to follow the Alternate-Day Diet.

Part One

HOW I ARRIVED AT THIS PLAN AND
WHY I KNOW IT WORKS

1.

Calorie Restriction: What It Means and Why You Probably Won't Do It

For the vast majority of dieters "calorie restriction" simply means reducing the number of calories they normally eat in order to lose weight, but for scientists investigating the potential benefits of restricting one's daily intake, that means allowing approximately 60 or 70 percent of what would be considered the "normal" caloric requirement to maintain weight while also maintaining optimal nutrition.

Probably the best-known and primary proponent of what its followers call Calorie Restriction with Optimal Nutrition, or CRON, was Roy Walford, mentioned in the introduction, who studied the phenomenon for many years at UCLA and produced significant evidence to support the theory that CRON could potentially extend human life to an average of 120 years.

PROOF THAT THIN IS BETTER

In 1935, Clive McCay, a well-known professor of nutrition at Cornell University, showed that rats fed a calorie-restricted diet lived longer, had less disease, had litters at later ages, and were much more active than the freely fed rats.

More recently, researchers have shown that restricting calories in lower life forms—including yeast, roundworms, and fruit flies—significantly prolonged their lives. In fact, Calorie Restriction, or CR, has been shown to prolong lifespan by amounts ranging up to 80 percent in virtually every species tested. Most important for humans, our close relative the rhesus monkey has been studied for more than fifteen years, and in every study the monkeys subjected to calorie restriction have appeared to be healthier than the freely fed controls.

Taking these studies a step further, Walford observed that by feeding rodents approximately 30 to 40 percent less than they would normally eat, they lost 10 to 25 percent of their normal body weight and lived 30 to 40 percent longer than their normal lifespan (that is, the lifespan of the normally fed control group). Although he was not specific about exactly how many calories any given individual should consume in a day, he did state that one ought to aim for a weight that is 10 to 25 percent below what was one's set point—the weight to which one's body naturally gravitates—during one's teenage years (assuming one was neither anorexic nor obese as a teenager) in order to achieve maximum metabolic efficiency and longevity. Weight loss, however, was considered incidental to the true goal of the diet, which was, first and foremost, to maximize health and longevity. And according to Walford, simply increasing one's activity level to burn additional calories, even if it resulted in weight loss, would not have the same health benefits as calorie restriction. (In fact, it is virtually impossible to increase one's activity level enough to achieve and maintain the degree of weight loss he recommends.) In truth, exercise alone, without calorie restriction, doesn't work for weight loss in general. It does, however, have other, important health-enhancing benefits, as you'll be learning in Chapter 6.

While most of Walford's testing was done on laboratory animals (as well as on himself), he had the unique opportunity to investigate the benefits of CRON on a group of human test subjects when he and seven fellow scientists entered Biosphere 2 in 1991 and discovered that their enclosed, self-sustaining environment was incapable of producing as much food as had been anticipated and would, therefore, be unable to supply the number of calories they were currently consuming. Although there was some initial discussion of simply abandoning Biosphere 2 altogether, Dr. Walford was able to persuade his fellow researchers that following a CRON diet for two years wouldn't harm them—and, in fact, could well improve their health and extend their life.

Since the group was dependent upon whatever food they could produce, their diet was consequently nutrient-dense—no calorie-dense and nutrient-deficient McDonald's or Dunkin' Donuts available. When the eight emerged after two years, they had all lost significant amounts of weight—the men on average about 18 percent and the women 10 percent of their pre-Biosphere body weight. They were all "thinner-than-thin," but there was no evidence that they were malnourished. Rather, tests indicated that they were actually nutritionally healthier than when they had gone in: Their cholesterol, triglyceride, fasting blood sugar, insulin, and blood pressure levels had all decreased. In fact, every one of the regularly measured laboratory markers showed results that were consistent with Dr. Walford's rodent studies in terms of their percentage of youthful values.

The evidence appears to be clear: According to Walter Willett, chairman of the Department of Nutrition at the Harvard School of Public Health, and a leading nutritional epidemiologist,

Calorie-Dense Versus Nutrient-Dense

Calorie-dense foods contain a high number of calories per unit of volume, meaning that you get a lot of calories for very little food. Nutrient-dense foods contain high levels of minerals, vitamins, phytonutrients, and other unknown factors that contribute to good health. Generally speaking, calorie-dense foods are nutrient-poor. (You may have heard them called "empty calories.") Nutrient-dense foods are usually lower in calories.

Humans have been genetically programmed to prefer foods that are high in fat and sugar, which are calorie-dense and not usually natural. Our obesity problem originates with our natural desire to consume these foods. The more readily they are available, the more we eat.

The opposite of calorie-dense foods are those with low calorie density. These are the foods on which many diets have been based. Among the most notable recent entries in the category of low-calorie-density diets is that recommended by Barbara Rolls in her book *Volumetrics*. The theory is that by eating a largely plant-based diet with a high water content, you will be able to eat more food while consuming fewer calories and will, therefore, feel full. One study done at Pennsylvania State University showed that dieters who ate a cup of soup or a salad before their meal consumed fewer total calories. Broth, fruits with high water content, nonstarchy vegetables, and lean proteins are part of this plan. In the Alternate-Day Diet the choice of foods recommended for both the "down days" and the "up days" is nutrient-dense and low-calorie.

the thinner we are, the healthier and longer-lived we will be. In the revised edition of his excellent book *Eat, Drink, and Be Healthy*, he states, "The lower and more stable your weight, the lower your chances of having or dying from a heart attack, stroke, or other type of cardiovascular disease; of developing high blood pressure, high cholesterol, or diabetes; of being diagnosed with postmenopausal breast cancer, cancer of the endometrium, colon, or kidney; or of being afflicted with some other chronic condition." And he goes on: "Keeping that number [your weight] in the healthy range is more important for long-term health than the types and the amounts of antioxidants in your food or the exact ratio of fats to carbohydrates." For example, being overweight doubles or triples your likelihood of heart disease. Even the effect of eating eight or more servings of fruits and vegetables a day compared with eating only 1.5 servings per day decreases the incidence of heart disease by only 25 percent and doesn't affect the overall incidence of cancer. Obesity and physical inactivity, on the other hand, may account for up to 30 percent of several major cancers including colon, endometrial, kidney, postmenopausal breast cancer, and cancer of the esophagus.

Although there are some studies that seem to indicate that being somewhat overweight is healthier than being very thin, life insurance companies—whose job it is to, in effect, bet on how long any given individual is likely to live—have used data collected over many years to conclude that death rates increase in people whose body mass index (BMI), a number that represents the relationship of height to weight, is higher than 21.

The primary source for these claims comes from studies in which groups of healthy people were followed for a period of approximately ten years. Their death rate was then examined in relation to their BMI. The studies showed that the number of

Calculate Your Own BMI

Your BMI is calculated by dividing your weight in pounds by your height in inches squared and then multiplying that number by 703.

deaths increased as BMI increased, meaning that the fatter you are, the more likely you are to die sooner.

In 2004, Luigi Fontana and his colleagues at Washington University in St. Louis published the first in a series of studies they did on members of the Calorie Restriction Society, proponents of restricting caloric intake to around 90 percent of recommended levels for weight maintenance. Their findings indicated that these people had lower risk factors for atherosclerosis, and the elasticity of their hearts was greater than those of the age- and gender-matched control group who ate a standard American diet. The average BMI of the control group was 26. In other

Healthspan Versus Lifespan

Many people who understand that Calorie Restriction prolongs lifespan say they don't want to simply "hang on" and experience the decrepitude of old age. But the good news is that studies indicate that older people who are in good health, as indicated by certain markers of aging, don't just live longer, they also have a longer healthspan—that is, the length of time they are actively mobile with good hearing, eyesight, and cognitive abilities.

words, those with the lower BMI had hearts that were functioning like the hearts of much younger people.

Interestingly the Calorie Restriction Society members studied by Fontana et al. had an average BMI of 19.7. If 21 is the

It Is Better to Be Thin and Eat "Bad" Food Than It Is to Be Overweight and Eat "Good" Food

Walter Willett states, "Your body weight is more important than the precise balance of healthy and unhealthy fats or whole grains versus refined carbohydrates or the number of servings of vegetables you eat."

In two major studies of the relationship between fruit and vegetable consumption and major chronic heart disease, stroke, cancer, and diabetes, the incidence of heart disease was 25 percent lower among those people who ate five or more servings compared with those who ate fewer than 1.5 servings. There was no significant overall reduction in cancer risk. In contrast, for a woman, having a BMI of 30 (the definition of obesity, 180 pounds for a 5'5" woman) is associated with a nearly 50 percent higher likelihood of dying and three times the incidence of heart disease than having a BMI of 21.

While I'm not advocating bad eating—in fact, it's just the opposite—it is important to understand that body weight supersedes other risk factors. Following the Alternate-Day Diet will minimize the impact of bad food for two reasons: First, because you will weigh less, and second, because it will activate a critical stress response you'll be learning about in Chapter 5.

optimal BMI according to the life insurance data collected by the Metropolitan Life Insurance Company, these CRON practitioners reduced their BMI by only 7 to 9 percent and yet they demonstrated marked health benefits! And, interestingly, none of the study participants in either group engaged in regular exercise. This and a host of other studies confirm the scientifically accepted wisdom that body weight is the most important factor in long-term survival. Exercise, dietary composition, serum cholesterol, and other risk factors are all of secondary importance.

Despite an abundance of compelling scientific evidence to support a healthier lifestyle, however, Americans are getting fatter. The National Center for Health Statistics reports that from 1962 to 2000 the number of obese Americans grew from 13 percent to 31 percent of the population. Furthermore, an article written by scientists at the Centers for Disease Control and published in the *Journal of the American Medical Association* indicated that in 2004 obesity was responsible for almost 112,000 deaths in the United States and probably more.

WHY CALORIE RESTRICTION ISN'T THE ANSWER

The health benefits of Calorie Restriction are irrefutable, but CRON is not a way of life that most people can embrace.

In early 2007 journalist Emily Yoffe interviewed Roy Walford's daughter, Lisa, now a leading proponent of CRON, for an article in the online publication *Slate.* Ms. Walford reported that she has a BMI of about 15. To get some perspective on what that means, Yoffe writes, "Spanish authorities banned from the runway models with BMIs of less than 18." Walford is about 5 feet tall and weighs 80 pounds. The article states that in her own book, coauthored with Brian Delaney, *The Longevity Diet*, she indicated that her usual breakfast consists of four walnuts, six almonds, and ten peanuts.

Lisa Walford has practiced Calorie Restriction for many years. An active, athletic yoga teacher, she has excellent HDL, total cholesterol, and triglyceride levels. In fact, by all indications she will live a long life. Although some very strong-willed individuals are able to achieve these goals, many, if not most, will fall by the wayside.

Aside from the question of whether most people would really want to have a BMI lower than that of most runway models, there is the issue of whether most people would want—much less be able—to spend their presumably increased lifespan consuming exactly twenty specific nuts for breakfast each day. Some critics have even suggested Calorie Restriction is an eating disorder, and somewhat wryly comment that while it may or may not prolong your life, it will certainly seem longer.

Calorie restrictors are exquisitely aware of exactly how many calories they are eating at all times. CRON, in other words, falls prey to one of the biggest stumbling blocks for any diet: It requires you to *constantly* think about the one thing you don't want to be thinking about: what you can and can't eat.

And interestingly, if "April's CR Diary," the online journal being kept by one member of the Calorie Restriction Society, is to be taken as typical, CRON followers (or at least a number of the women among them) appear to remain extremely focused on and unhappy with their weight—perhaps because they're frustrated at not being able to achieve Roy Walford's "ideal" of maintaining a body weight that's 10 to 25 percent below the standard optimal BMI of 21.

In the final analysis, however, the major reason why daily

Calorie Restriction is not viable for most people is that so few people are able to maintain *any* level of calorie reduction over time. Surrounded by an increasing abundance of tasty, affordable food, we seem to be unable to restrain ourselves, and, as a result, people are getting fatter. And the problem is by no means limited to the United States. Other developed countries are witnessing similar increases in obesity as they move away from

French Women Do Get Fat

The French have long prided themselves on being the thinnest population in the world. But now a parliamentary report states that their rate of obesity is increasing even more quickly than that of Americans and may match it by the year 2020.

While I certainly agree with the cultural and thoughtful approach to food described by Mireille Guiliano in *French Women Don't Get Fat,* the reality is that even the French are getting fatter.

The average French family dinner, which lasted 88 minutes twenty-five years ago, now lasts 38 minutes, and the French are becoming more American in their ways of eating in front of the TV, on the telephone, and when by themselves.

Of particular note is that McDonald's is more profitable in France than anywhere else in Europe. Sales have increased 42 percent over the past five years, and some 1.2 million French, or 2 percent of the population, eat there every day. (By comparison, in the United States, 5 percent of the population eats at McDonald's on a daily basis.)

a nutrient-rich to a calorie-dense diet. Even French women do get fat.

In fact the Chinese, the Russians, Eskimos from Greenland, and sub-Saharan Africans are all getting fatter, as is every other population when economic conditions improve and there is increased access to cheaper food. In fact, there are now as many overweight as malnourished people in the world.

I know myself well enough to understand that daily Calorie Restriction won't work for me, and if you've been battling weight problems, it's probably not for you either. Like me, however, you may well be able to enjoy the same health benefits by following the Alternate-Day Diet, which is more compatible with—and forgiving of—human nature and allows you to continue enjoying most of the pleasures of eating.

2.

The Truths About Dieting

A fter observing my own and many other people's relationship to food over many years, I have come up with a list of the "dietary truths" that I consider to be self-evident. While I don't claim that these are revolutionary or even original thoughts, I do believe that it's important to list them here, clearly and explicitly, because understanding and accepting them will help you to understand why you need to have a specific, practical plan to help you respond to and combat them.

1. Humans have evolved with a preference for foods with a high calorie density and to eat whenever food is available.

As our species evolved and food was scarce, survival (evolution) favored those who ate the most and who ate foods that were high in calories and, therefore, provided the most energy. Over the centuries, these behaviors have been programmed into our DNA.

2. The cheaper and more available food becomes, the more we will eat and the fatter we will be.

There are many theories offering alternative biological explanations for obesity, but none, other than the change in the food environment, reasonably explain the huge rise in obesity we are currently witnessing.

According to *The Economics of Obesity: A Report on the Workshop Held at USDA's Economic Research Service*, by Tomas Philipson, Carolanne Dai, Lorens Helmchen, and Jayachandran N. Variyam, the worldwide long-term increase in obesity is clearly correlated with technological improvements that reduce the cost of food.

Having historically survived by eating as much as we could whenever we could, we are now genetically programmed to do that. The more primitive, nonrational part of our brain (often termed the "reptile brain") is constantly telling us to eat. The difference between us and our ancestors is that we now have an endless supply of relatively low-cost food always available. At this point each of us is, figuratively speaking, a great crocodile swimming through a sea of tempting foods that are constantly saying, "Eat me, eat me!" and too often we find that the rational control part of our brain is unable to overcome the temptation.

In *The Omnivore's Dilemma*, author Michael Pollan blames the increase in obesity on the collusion between the federal government and agribusiness that has created increasingly cheaper commodities such as corn. But the fact of the matter is that all food commodities have gotten enormously cheaper (and proportionately cheaper than other consumer goods), as has everything else in our consumer society, in the past fifty years. The incredible success of our free-market economy has increased the

Your Reptile Brain on Junk Food

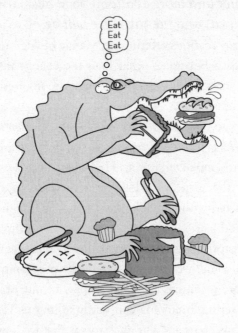

efficiency of production across the board and is responsible for the lower costs of *everything*, not just foods.

To compound the problem, the commercial food industry is constantly bombarding us with messages designed to get us to eat their products, which translates to an incessant demand that we eat more and more. In fact, according to Brian Wansink, director of the Cornell University Food and Brand Lab and author of *Mindless Eating*, each of us makes more than 200 food-related decisions every day, mostly without even being conscious we're making them.

3. Our appetite-control mechanism is broken.

The most reasonable explanation for the explosion of obesity throughout the world is that the mechanism controlling our internal appetite-signaling device is broken. Although the terms "hunger" and "appetite" are often used interchangeably, we can no longer differentiate one from the other. We have a desire to eat when we see something tasty (or simply when we just think about eating something we like) whether or not we are actually hungry. In fact, many of us no longer know what hunger feels like because we haven't allowed ourselves to become hungry in years.

In a May 2007 article in *Time* magazine, "The Science of Appetite," Jeffrey Kluger wrote: "Somewhere in your brain, there's a cupcake circuit. How it works is not entirely clear, and you couldn't see it even if you knew where to look. But it's there all the same—and it's a powerful thing. You didn't pop out of the womb prewired for cupcakes, but long ago, early in your babyhood, you got your first taste of one, and instantly a series of sensory, metabolic and neurochemical fireworks went off.

"The mesolimbic region in the center of your brain—the area that processes pleasure—lit up. . . . Your midbrain filed away a simple, primal, unconscious idea: *Cupcakes are good*. A lifetime love affair—perhaps pleasant, perhaps tortured—began."

Kluger then goes on to discuss the many biochemical mechanisms by which we humans regulate hunger. Among them is a hormone called ghrelin, discovered in 1999. It was dubbed the hunger hormone, because when ghrelin is produced in the gut we want to eat. It is designed to be released in response to meal schedules, but according to some theories, Kluger says, ghrelin is also released by "the mere sight or smell of food." In other words, our appetite is stimulated whether or not we're hungry, whether or not it's actually time for us to eat.

Scientists are diligently looking into what it is that makes us hungry and what makes us feel full, but whatever chemicals may be contributing or used to control the increase in human obesity, the pleasure principle always seems to be at work. According to Barbara Rolls, of Pennsylvania State University's College of Health and Human Development, one of the things that gives us pleasure is variety in our meals. Loading up on one particular food, she says, may satisfy our desire for that particular nutrient, but it will still leave us craving something else. Rolls calls this "sensory-specific satiety" and relates it to the fact that even after a large and satisfying meal we, more often than not, can still find room for dessert.

Kluger concludes his article by saying, "We may always be pleasure-seeking creatures, intoxicated by the very experience of food—with its colors and textures and notes of flavor." And if that's so, "The same human brain that invented the food court and the supermarket must now develop ways to control how we use them."

THE EMOTIONAL EATING COMPONENT

Eating for pleasure can readily sabotage our efforts to control consumption. There is significant evidence to show that much of our overeating or eating when we're not really hungry is triggered by an emotional component. Just as Pavlov's dogs were trained to eat at the sign of a bell, we more or less automatically eat at mealtimes. But emotions may also trigger that Pavlovian response. We may eat when we're stressed, sad, anxious, angry, frustrated, or just plain bored. Without being consciously aware

High-Fat, High-Sugar Foods Disrupt Our Appetite Control Mechanism

Under normal circumstances, our brain accurately senses our nutrient needs and sends signals to our body that automatically control our energy balance so that we consume almost exactly the same amount every day, thereby maintaining stable body weight.

The regulation of food intake is a complex feedback system affected by environment and psychological factors, but that system is made dysfunctional when we eat foods rich in fat and sugar.

These foods activate the brain's "reward" system, which means that we are eating not because we need the calories for energy but because our brain is responding to the food in the same way it responds to an addictive drug. Levels of brain substances that make us feel good—such as dopamine, serotonin, and endogenous opiates—rise, and because of this we eat longer and more ("going back for seconds") than we normally would.

At the same time, these foods blunt the satiety signals that would normally tell us it's time to stop eating.

Over time, we adapt to high-fat, high-sugar foods by increasing the amount we eat in order to get that mental "fix." It feels like we're just satisfying our hunger, but from the standpoint of brain function, we are reacting as if we were enjoying the effects of a drug "high."

of what we're *really* hungry for, we attempt to quiet the emotional turmoil with food. And the foods we tend to eat in those situations are usually calorie-dense, nutrient-deficient "comfort" foods. Chocolate, for example, has been shown to increase brain levels of the neurotransmitter serotonin, which is the same chemical that is increased by many antidepressant medications. Sugary foods create an upsurge in blood sugar that gives us a quick energy boost. Then, because eating those foods does, in fact, make us feel better in the short term, we turn to them again and again, much as a drug addict turns to his opiate of choice to escape negative emotions.

Emotional eating can also be a learned behavior. Perhaps your mother taught you to associate eating with pleasure. She may have rewarded you with food for good behavior. Or perhaps you grew up in a large family where sitting around the table at dinnertime was an enjoyable part of your day. Conversely, your mother may have restricted your access to sweets, and you learned to associate eating candy with guilty pleasure. Maybe you were punished for bad behavior by not being allowed to eat dessert.

Whatever the reason, the problem with emotional eating is twofold. Eating unconsciously doesn't solve the underlying problems that triggered our desire to eat in the first place. And because we're normally unaware of *why* we're eating at any particular moment, it can lead to serious and potentially unhealthy weight gain.

EVERYBODY WILL BE FAT

If we don't exercise our free will to overcome the base reptilian thinking patterns—to eat whenever and wherever food is available—and to control the primal urge to seek the pleasure of food, in another thirty years all but perhaps the lucky 10 percent of us who can eat without restriction and not gain weight will be fat.

4. All diets work. All diets fail.

According to a study conducted by Michael Dansinger of Tufts–New England Medical Center in Boston, *adherence* to a weight-loss plan—any plan—is more important for success than what the specific plan might be. On the other side of the coin, Bärbel Knäuper, associate professor of psychology at McGill University in Montreal, states that the number-one cause of dieting failure is setting goals that are not realistic.

Most overweight people have attempted to lose weight and many have been successful for a time. Even the most outrageous-sounding diet will work as long as we remain conscious of what we are eating and stick with it, but all diets will fail eventually unless we devise a plan that can be followed indefinitely. That is, we have to find a way to beat the statistics that indicate that close to 100 percent of those who succeed in losing weight will regain it within five years.

Anyone will lose weight on whatever diet they choose to follow so long as it results in reducing total calorie intake. When it comes to weight loss, nutrient balance isn't really the issue. Whether we restrict fat or carbohydrates or protein, the bottom line is to take in fewer calories than we expend. But the overwhelming body of evidence indicates that any form of constant daily restriction will not work because we simply can't stick with it.

When we start a new diet we develop a feeling of euphoria that helps us to stay on the program and not feel hungry, but gradually that feeling goes away. Eventually we'll feel frustrated, hungry, deprived, bored, or just plain disappointed because we've lost weight and our life hasn't radically changed for the better. (We've set unrealistic goals not only for our weight loss but for lifestyle issues that accompany it.) When these feelings occur, we stop following the diet and, almost inevitably, regain the weight we lost.

5. No diet will work without a plan that overcomes our inclination to eat whenever and whatever food is available.

The extent of the obesity problem today is self-evident. Most of us are overweight and it is reasonable to assume that most of us don't want to be. The "natural history" of body weight in the current environment was clearly demonstrated in a ten-year community-based volunteer study conducted by Harvard surgeon George L. Blackburn and his colleagues.

In the course of the study, one group of people substituted a meal-replacement shake or nutrition bar for one or two meals a day while the control group ate normally. Those who used the shake experienced a sustained weight loss of 6.2 pounds over ten years while the control group gained 26.6 pounds, an average of 2.5 pounds per year, creating a differential between the two groups of 33 pounds over all.

Logically one would have to assume that many if not all the people who ate normally were making some effort to control their weight since they were participating in a study. If so, they were typical victims of their genes, their emotions, and our food-rich environment. To me, therefore, these results indicate that we need to have a specific self-monitoring plan (such as one that uses a meal-replacement shake) in order to avoid becoming fatter over time. Simply wanting to lose weight—or not gain—over time requires such a plan, without which no amount of will-power will be enough.

6. The only diet that will continue to work over the long haul is one that involves a long-term strategy.

Recent studies that compared different kinds of diets—Atkins, Weight Watchers, Dean Ornish—show only minor differences in the amount of weight lost at the end of one year, indicating that all diets will work in the short term. But experience shows they will all fail in the long term.

There are members of the National Weight Control Registry—established in 1994—who are on record as having been able to maintain a weight loss of over 30 pounds for at least five years. And another group, which was studied by James W. Anderson, MD, and colleagues at the University of Kentucky, involved very obese people who had lost 100 pounds and maintained a weight loss of 66 pounds for a period of five years.

Variety may be the spice of life but there is ample science showing that the greater the variety in a diet, the higher the calorie intake. The National Weight Control Registry partici-pants have very low levels of variety. Monotony in flavor is help-ful in reducing how much you eat. *The Shangri-La Diet* and *The Flavor Point Diet* are based on this principle.

I suggest that you find five recipes of low-calorie-density food that you enjoy and can eat over and over.

While these "maintainers" are still in the minority, a key to their success appears to be a shift from a short-term diet mentality to a long-term strategy. My extensive experience with dieters is that the Alternate-Day Diet lends itself to a maintenance mentality, because not only does it take into account the self-evident dietary truths, it also avoids a feeling of deprivation on a daily basis.

3.

The Alternate-Day Advantage

Ironically, I have to thank a group of rodents that had been genetically altered to gorge for helping me find a way to overcome the gorging DNA that's hardwired into my reptilian brain.

THE LESSON OF MATTSON'S MICE

In 2003 I read about an experiment, described briefly in the Introduction, done by Mark Mattson and his colleagues at the National Institute on Aging. That experiment had, in turn, been inspired by a previous study completed by Mattson's colleague Donald Ingram. Ingram looked at two groups of mice from the time they were weaned until the time they died. One group was given free access to all the food they wanted on a daily basis, while the second group was also fed freely but only every other day. The group fed on alternate days was found to live an average of 30 percent longer than the group that was fed freely on a daily basis.

Based on Ingram's findings, Mattson took the study one step further. Using three groups of the same strain of mice (which had been genetically altered to gorge when given free access to food), he and his colleagues fed two groups exactly as Ingram had fed his. The third group was fed a daily diet that was restricted to approximately 40 percent of their normal caloric intake.

More Than Just Weight Loss

At the end of the twenty-week study, the group that had been fed a restricted diet on a daily basis lost weight, and tests also showed that their glucose and insulin levels were reduced, while insulin sensitivity and "stress resistance" were increased compared with the group that was fed freely every day. Lower glucose and insulin levels are known indicators of longer lifespan and are associated with a reduction in heart disease and diabetes. This was certainly not surprising, because it replicated Ingram's findings, and, as we've discussed, dietary restriction had already been shown in other studies to positively affect health and longevity. What really caught my attention, however, was that the mice who were fed only on alternate days—even though they gorged on the days they were fed freely and did not lose weight—had levels that were as good or better than those who were restricted on a daily basis.

Another indicator of health and longevity is the degree to which the central nervous system is able to resist and recover from the stresses to which it is subjected throughout life. In humans, the resilience of the central nervous system is an indicator of how people will react to brain disorders such as stroke and Alzheimer's disease and their ability to resist the effects of environmental toxins. Mattson examined the ability of the central

Resistance, Resilience, and Recovery

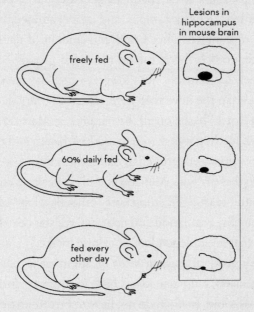

Lesions in hippocampus in mouse brain

freely fed

60% daily fed

fed every other day

Following several weeks on one of three diets, mice were injected with an excitotoxin that would mimic the kind of neurological damage caused by diseases such as stroke, Alzheimer's, or Parkinson's. Mice fed every other day, while eating enough on their feeding day to maintain the same weight as the freely fed mice, showed distinctly smaller lesions in the hippocampus than either of the other groups, indicating that alternate-day feeding led to increased health and potential longevity over either free feeding or daily restriction.

nervous system to resist stress in each of the three groups of mice. To do this he subjected the mice to an artificially created brain injury by injecting a toxic chemical (kainate) into a portion of the brain called the hippocampus, and later examined the extent of the area of damage. Once again, the amount of damage was markedly reduced in both calorie-restricted groups compared with the freely fed controls, but the every-other-day-fed mice had less damage than the mice that were restricted every day.

In other words, based on all the parameters Mattson studied, alternate-day feeding was shown to increase health and potential longevity to a greater degree than daily restriction.

Based on these results, Mattson and his colleagues concluded that intermittent fasting (feeding every other day) has "beneficial effects on glucose regulation and neuronal resistance to injury in these mice that are independent of caloric intake."

What this groundbreaking study meant to me is that animals (and by extension, humans) do not have to restrict caloric intake on a daily basis and, further, do not have to be thin to be in good health.

HOW ELSE CAN ALTERNATE-DAY DIETING IMPROVE YOUR HEALTH?

If calorie restriction, especially every-other-day feeding, promotes good cardiac and central nervous system health, what else might it do? Might it also help prevent cancer?

Marc Hellerstein, an endocrinologist at the University of California at Berkeley, demonstrated the effect of alternate-day feeding on the rate at which the cells of various tissues divided (proliferated) in a group of mice. The rate at which cells divide and proliferate is an indicator of the likelihood of developing cancer. Dr. Hellerstein's experiment showed that the rate at which skin cells, breast gland cells, and T-lymphocytes proliferated was markedly reduced within just two weeks in mice fed every other day, even though the total number of calories these mice received was not substantially reduced. These findings could be considered an indication of potentially profound cancer prevention benefits for human beings.

Another study conducted in France by Olivier Descamps and colleagues using a group of middle-aged mice that were genetically predisposed to be at high risk for developing lymphoma also demonstrated that alternate-day feeding protected against cancer. Over the four-month period of the study, *not one* of the mice being fed on alternate days developed lymphoma, while 33 percent of the control group did. In addition, the researchers found that oxidative damage to the mitochondria (the principal energy source of the cell), a basic indicator of aging, was significantly decreased in the alternate-day-fed mice. The investigators concluded that "the efficacy of alternate fasting did not really depend on calorie restriction," and that "alternate fasting could exert a beneficial antioxidant effect and a modulation of the oxidative stress associated with aging."

OXIDATIVE STRESS AND AGING

In 1954, a young physician named Denham Harman proposed an idea that changed the way scientists thought about how we age. His Free Radical Theory of Aging said that a side effect of oxygen metabolism in our bodies is the production of chemicals that gradually damage our cells, protein, and DNA, ultimately resulting in death. This damage, caused by so-called free radicals, is known as oxidative stress. His theory was not initially taken seriously within the medical community, but over time, medical research has caught up with Harman, and it is now widely accepted that the damage done by oxidative stress is the primary cause of aging in humans.

When apples turn brown, butter turns rancid, or iron rusts, they are "aging" and exhibiting the results of exposure to oxidative damage. Our bodies may not exhibit oxidative damage externally, but it is there just the same. Our bodies are made up of atoms and molecules, each of which contains one or more pairs of electrons. Over time, normal metabolism, mainly in the mitochondria, causes the formation of "free radicals," which are atoms that have lost one electron. Free radicals are unstable and attempt to complete their structure and regain stability by "stealing" an electron from another, neighboring molecule. That, of course, prompts the molecule that's been "robbed" of its electron to do the same thing, causing even further damage. The products of free-radical damage are like sludge that builds up in the cells, causing malfunctions and, ultimately, stress that is sufficient to cause the cell to die.

The same process also causes inflammation on the cellular level that, in turn, causes more oxidative damage. Both inflammation and oxidative stress have been shown to be associated with a number of chronic illnesses of aging, including atherosclerosis, arthritis, Type 2 diabetes, and Alzheimer's disease.

Oxidative stress is reduced by both daily and alternate-day calorie restriction, possibly as a result of reduced oxygen consumption.

Telomeres and Oxidative Damage

Telomeres are the ends of the chromosomes that become shorter as we age. This is because imperfect replication of the telomere occurs when cells divide, and some of the DNA is lost with each cell division. Eventually the cell cannot divide without damage to critical parts of the DNA, and it becomes senescent (not yet dead but not functioning normally), necroses (dies), or undergoes apoptosis (cell suicide).

We know that oxidative damage caused by free radicals is associated with shorter telomeres. Thus at a given age, those who undergo more oxidative stress will have shorter telomeres. People with shorter telomeres are 3 times more likely to die of heart disease and 8.5 times more likely to die of infectious disease.

Chronic inflammation means that white blood cells replicate more quickly, which, presumably, results in shorter telomeres. It seems reasonable to postulate, therefore, that people with chronic inflammation would have shorter telomeres at an earlier age, which would lead to premature cell senescence, necrosis, or apoptosis and earlier onset of chronic diseases of aging.

Because of its powerful anti-inflammatory effects, the Alternate-Day Diet will reduce the chronic oxidative damage and premature telomere shortening involved in such diseases as atherosclerosis, and would prolong life.

Oxidative Stress and Disease

Oxidative stress has been associated with some 250 diseases and with virtually all diseases of aging.

- **Atherosclerosis:** LDL cholesterol is deposited in the artery wall. Then free radicals "oxidize" the LDL by causing it to lose an electron, which makes the oxidized LDL irritating to the tissues and causes inflammation. This inflammation results in the formation of plaque in the wall of the artery, which obstructs the opening of the artery and eventually blocks the flow of blood.
- **Arthritis** is caused by oxidative damage in the joints. Inflammation causes increased oxidative damage.
- **Alzheimer's disease:** The first event in Alzheimer's disease is oxidative injury to the neuron, leading to the formation of a neurofibrillar tangle and deposits of beta-amyloid plaque.
- **Cancer:** An early step in the formation of cancer is often free-radical damage to the DNA that causes cells to mutate or change.
- **Diabetes mellitus:** Oxidative stress causes insulin resistance, the major contributor to Type 2 diabetes.

Low levels of oxidative stress are probably essential to reaching old age by preventing disease. At least two studies have shown lower levels of oxidative stress in individuals one hundred years old than in individuals seventy years old, suggesting that a low level of oxidative stress may be required to reach advanced ages.

How Free Radicals and Inflammation Cause Heart Disease and Stroke

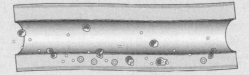

Elevated blood LDL cholesterol is deposited in the artery wall and is oxidized by free radicals, producing inflammation.

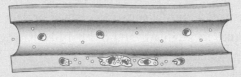

White blood cells ingest oxidized LDL, forming large foam cells. A pimple begins to form.

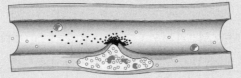

The pimple breaks, spewing inflammatory material into the bloodstream. This leads to clot formation.

By reducing inflammation and free-radical damage, Alternate-Day dieting helps prevent heart disease and stroke.

WHAT IF HUMANS ATE LESS OFTEN?

A number of studies suggest that it would be healthier to eat less often than most of us do—which is typically three times a day. One such study, which looked at people who were fasting for 12 to 14 hours during the thirty days of Ramadan, indicated that good cholesterol levels went up and there was a reduction in inflammatory chemicals (cytokines) in the bloodstream, with no weight loss.

Mark Mattson also performed a study of humans who were fed all their daily calories during a single four-hour period. In this case, the study subjects lost only 3 pounds over the six-month study, but they showed a 4.6-pound reduction in body fat, which meant that they had *gained* 1.4 pounds in lean muscle tissue. This may seem like a modest change, but reducing body fat by almost 5 pounds means a lot less inflammation is occurring. In this case, however, the study participants complained of greater hunger than when they ate regularly and did not like having to eat all their food in this limited period.

Both these studies, however, beg the question "Would we benefit from alternate-day calorie restriction?"

ALTERNATE-DAY CALORIE RESTRICTION BENEFITS PEOPLE TOO

The medical literature contains only one long-term study of humans that is described as an experiment in calorie restriction performed in a controlled setting with good nutrition. Published in a Spanish medical journal, *Revista Clinica Española*, in 1956, this study was conducted by Eduardo Arias Vallejo on a group of healthy male and female residents of the Residencia Geriatrica de San José, an old-age home in Madrid. At the time, Vallejo was the medical director of the residence and later became president of the Sociedad Española de Patología Digestiva (Spanish Society of Digestive Pathology).

When I read the original version of the study, however, it became clear that there was no overall calorie reduction involved. Rather, the test subjects were experiencing alternate-day restriction, eating less than their normal caloric requirement on one day and more on the next, so that on average their caloric intake was not actually restricted at all. There was also a control group who were fed "normally" every day.

Before we could analyze the study correctly, however, my colleagues and I needed to know the average daily calorie consumption of an elderly Spanish person in 1956. We consulted height and body weight data for Spaniards in the 1950s and determined that it would have been about 1,600 calories per day averaging both men and women.

On the low-calorie day the study subjects were given a liter of milk and 500 grams of fresh fruit, which we estimated to be approximately 900 to 950 calories, or 56 percent of the approximately 1,600 they would normally eat. Vallejo states that on the "up days" the diet subjects consumed 2,300 calories. Presumably, on those days they were allowed to eat as much as they wanted, and the 2,300-calorie figure was probably derived from adding up what they took on their trays at mealtime as recorded by the kitchen staff.

Based on these figures, the "restricted" study subjects were actually compensating for their 900-calorie down days by consuming 144 percent of normal daily caloric intake on their up days, so that their up and down days averaged out to a "normal" 1,600 calories per day. In other words, there was no overall reduction in calories at all.

Although others have interpreted this study to show that the diet subjects were receiving 35 percent *less* than their normal calorie intake, their interpretation is based on a mistranslation that led them to conclude that the control subjects (those who were not on the diet) were consuming 2,300 calories daily. But Vallejo does not state that in his article. He simply states that the control group was fed the same food as the diet group on a daily basis (meaning they would have taken food that totaled 1,600 calories on average per day).

For comparison, the most recent Dietary Guidelines for Americans produced by the U.S. Department of Health and Human Services recommend an average calorie consumption for sedentary people over age fifty-one of 1,800 calories per day (men 2,000 and women 1,600). These modern-day Americans are both taller and heavier, with a BMI of 26 to 27, than Spaniards born in the 1870s and 1880s. The point is, even by today's standards, 2,300 calories would be much too high an estimate of average daily calorie need.

Unfortunately, Dr. Vallejo did not comment on the body weight of his subjects, presumably because it didn't change. But if their caloric intake had been reduced by 35 percent, as suggested by some authors, these elderly people would have lost 80 pounds in the first year of the study.

Frankly, my colleague Dr. Laub and I find it impossible to imagine that Dr. Vallejo, the nuns of St. Joseph who ran the old-age home, the patients themselves, or their families would have permitted such systematic starvation to occur.

The study lasted three years, after which the two groups were compared. The diet group spent a total of 123 days in the hospital, while the control group spent a total of 219, and there were six deaths among the dieters as opposed to thirteen among the control group. In short, the diet reduced the likelihood of severe illness and death by half, as compared with the controls.

How Much Longer Would Vallejo's Subjects Live?

Normally, in animal studies, the lengthening of lifespan in calorie-restricted animals is expressed as a percentage increase over that of a control group. In other words, all the animals in the study die at various ages, which are plotted on a graph like the one below. All the animals are alive as shown on the y-axis at the beginning of the study, and as time passes on the x-axis all of them die eventually. The difference is that the calorie-restricted animals live about 40 percent longer—that is, they die at later ages. For example, a mouse species that lives 2 years on average would live 2.8 years when calorie restricted.

SURVIVAL CURVE

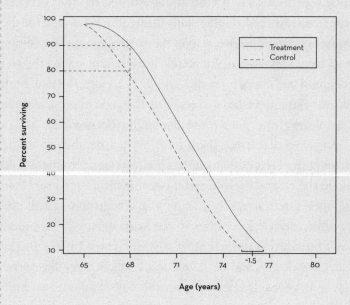

If we reconstruct the mortality curve for those in the Vallejo study, we see that these human subjects followed the same pattern. In 1957 the average life expectancy in Spain was 69.7 years. When we plot the death rate for the two groups, we see a shift to the right of approximately eighteen months for the diet group, indicating a 50 percent prolongation of life among those who followed the diet over the entire three-year period. This is only an educated guess and pertains only to the duration of the study, but it is in the same general range as the effect of calorie restriction on other species.

What Caused These Deaths?

The biggest differential between the two groups in the Vallejo study was in the number of deaths from heart disease. There were three myocardial infarctions (heart attacks) among the diet group as opposed to five among the control group. In addition, there were four cases of congestive heart failure among the control group and none in the diet group. Therefore, the total number of deaths from heart disease in the control group (9) was three times greater than those among the diet group (3).

As we've discussed, there have been a number of studies showing the profound ameliorative effects of intermittent feeding on the central nervous system in animals. In the heart there are specialized fibers constituting a conduction system that transmits electrical impulses to the heart muscle in an orderly way to produce a normal heart rhythm. These fibers function much like nerves, and Dr. Laub and I believe that, like nerves, they were probably affected by the up-day down-day pattern of the Vallejo study. Because many deaths from myocardial infarction are due to abnormal heart rhythms, which would be minimized if the conduction fibers were healthier, we speculate that the primary protective effect the diet had on heart attacks as well as on congestive heart failure resulted from its beneficial effect on this conduction system.

Looking at the figures for cancer deaths—two in each group—it would initially appear that the diet did not protect against cancer. But cancer is a disease that may be present in the body for years before it becomes apparent, and the three-year duration of the study might have been too short a time to have had an impact on the development of the disease. In fact, as we have seen, other studies do show a strong protective effect against cancer from calorie restriction in animals, and there is also extensive human data to show that people who eat less have lower rates of cancer.

Finally, among the nonfatal illnesses for which the subjects in the Vallejo study were treated, there were eight cases of bronchitis (an infectious disease) in the control group and three in the diet group. My own observation has been that there is a marked reduction in the incidence and severity of upper respiratory infection among people following the Alternate-Day Diet, and, in fact, members of the Calorie Restriction Society report that they have many fewer colds than they did before they began to practice Calorie Restriction.

Calorie-restricted animals have also been shown to have a reduction in infectious disease, which appears to result from a healthier immune response. For example, although the number of circulating lymphocytes (a type of white blood cell that defends against infection and tumors) in calorie-restricted animals is reduced by one-third, the lymphocytes are more effective than those in unrestricted animals.

WHAT IF YOU DON'T GORGE?

In both Mattson's mouse study and Vallejo's human study, test subjects ate more than their normal calorie requirement on the days when their feeding was not restricted, and yet they still showed significant health benefits as compared with their control groups. When I considered this evidence, it seemed clear to me that alternate-day feeding, even without calorie reduction or significant weight loss, could improve health and extend longevity in much the same way as daily restriction.

More recently, there has been one additional study done on humans subjected to alternate-day fasting. In this study, conducted in early 2005 by the world-renowned metabolic researcher Eric Ravussin and his associates at the Pennington Biomedical Research Center in Baton Rouge, Louisiana, sixteen people of normal weight (eight men and eight women) were put on an alternate-day fasting regimen for three weeks. On the fast day, they were allowed to consume only calorie-free soft drinks, tea, coffee, and sugar-free gum. On the alternate days they could eat whatever they wished. At the end of the study they had all lost weight, indicating, according to the researchers, "that the subjects were unable to consume enough food on the feasting days to maintain their weight." But the researchers also noted that "a prolonged schedule of fasting and feasting would be marred by aversive subjective states (e.g., hunger and irritability), which would likely limit the ability of most individuals to sustain this eating pattern." In other words, they were saying that no one would eat that way willingly.

When I first conceived of the Alternate-Day Diet in 2003, I had independently decided that most people would be unlikely to tolerate a down day of less than 20 percent of their normal calorie intake for any substantial period of time, so I was pleased to note that Ravussin concluded his article by saying that "adding a small meal (10 to 20 percent of caloric needs) to the fasting day may make alternate-day fasting more acceptable in all populations."

I had asked myself, "What would happen if one severely restricted calories on alternate days without actually fasting and *didn't* overeat or gorge on the up days?"

Using myself as a test group of one, I put myself on a diet of 20 percent of normal calories on alternate days, figuring that this would be restrictive enough to trigger the health benefits seen by Mattson and Vallejo without actually fasting. On the days when I wasn't restricting, I ate as I normally would. Initially, I made little effort to follow a healthy diet. In fact, I didn't hesitate to eat McDonald's fries or (my personal favorite) Popeye's spicy fried chicken.

Interestingly, I discovered that I wasn't excessively hungry and wasn't tempted to overeat on the up days to "make up for" the days when I was eating very little. And I found it relatively easy to muster the willpower to comply with my self-imposed regimen, because I knew that I'd never be depriving myself for more than one day at a time.

As I've already said, I lost 35 pounds within the first 11 weeks of my new diet, and other markers of health, including my cholesterol and triglyceride levels, improved and have remained so.

MY PERSONAL WEIGHT-LOSS EPIPHANY

What started as a personal experiment to measure the possible health benefits of an alternate-day calorie-restriction pattern became something else. I eventually realized that alternate-day dieting was the only way I had ever been able to lose weight and maintain the weight loss. Since May 2003, I have personally put many hundreds of people on the diet, and thousands of others who learned about the diet have shared their Alternate-Day experiences online in a variety of blogs.

4.

The Asthma Study

When I first put myself on the Alternate-Day Diet, I found, to my surprise, that within just two weeks the arthritis I'd had in my shoulder for more than five years improved tremendously. I was so pleased with the results that I told a good friend of mine what I'd been doing. Lenny, a fifty-seven-year-old trial lawyer, was naturally a skeptical guy, but he decided to try it himself. For some time, he'd been plagued by a painful heel spur that, according to his orthopedist, would only be helped by surgery, and, much as Lenny loved a good challenge, that option wasn't one he wanted to accept. Shortly after starting the diet, he took his family on a ski vacation in Sun Valley, Idaho. On their first day there he tried to hike up a 6,000-foot mountain with his kids but had to stop after 200 feet because of the intense pain in his foot. Ten days later, on the last day of their vacation, he hiked the entire mountain with no pain at all. Lenny was convinced. He continued to follow the diet, eventually lost 25 pounds, and is still following his own modified version of the Alternate-Day plan. He's kept the weight off and hasn't had any recurrence of the problem with his heel.

My own outcome and Lenny's—particularly in terms of the rapidity with which they occurred—were fascinating to me, and I started to put some of my patients on the diet. Marla was the classic example of a woman with a lovely face hidden in layers of fat. She came to see me about a cosmetic procedure that, as I explained to her, I couldn't perform because I was afraid that her weight would put her at serious risk. She was 5 feet, 4 inches tall and weighed 213 pounds. Coincidentally, she was also using three different types of inhaled bronchodilators for asthma twice a day. She wasn't in denial about her problem, just incredibly frustrated by her past attempts to lose weight, and she asked me what kind of diet I'd recommend. When I told her about the Alternate-Day Diet and its apparent health benefits, she was more than willing to try it. Before she began, we drew blood to measure her insulin and serum lipid levels and determined that she would use 400 calories in the form of a commercial meal-replacement shake to control her calorie intake on the down day.

After three weeks on the diet, Marla was using her inhalers only once a day, and after six weeks she was off them entirely. I, along with Marla and her pulmonologist, was amazed. Although she did lose weight—she was down to 198 pounds after six weeks—the weight loss alone wasn't significant enough to account for such a drastic pulmonary improvement.

In addition, her insulin levels were initially so high that she was at very high risk for developing diabetes. I tested her insulin level at two, four, six, and eight weeks. It remained at 30 micro units per milliliter of blood serum through six weeks, and then at eight weeks it suddenly dropped to 10 and continued to decrease over the next four months from 10 to 8 to 3 to 1 micro unit per milliliter, even though her weight had stabilized at 178 pounds. What's particularly interesting about these findings is that even though Marla was still overweight, her insulin levels continued to improve.

After a while, Marla admitted to me that while she was still on the diet, she was eating closer to 30 or 35 percent than 20 percent of her normal calorie requirement on the down days as well as more than she had been during her first few weeks on the diet on the up days. So even this less restrictive approach to Alternate-Day dieting was sufficient to continue improving her insulin response—an outcome that replicated Mattson's findings, in which insulin levels decreased the most in the mice who were fed on alternate days even though they didn't lose weight.

After eight months Marla called me one evening in the throes of a severe asthma attack. When I asked what had happened, she confessed that she'd gone off the diet three weeks before because she wanted to see if it really was curing her asthma. I guess she was convinced, because she went back on the diet and had the same improvement she experienced the first time.

Would It Work for Others as Well?

Along with my own experience and that of my friend, Marla's improvement seemed to indicate a high degree of anti-inflammatory benefit from following a diet based on alternate-day calorie restriction. At that point, I was eager to test for myself, under controlled circumstances, whether it was a feasible method of dietary restriction that could improve the lives of a specific population with observable health issues.

To do that, my colleagues and I recruited a single group of ten overweight people who had stable, moderate, persistent asthma with daily symptoms. Our goal was to determine whether they would adhere to a diet providing 20 percent or less of their normal calorie intake on alternate days, and whether the diet would affect their weight and/or the severity of their symptoms.

There were three reasons for choosing asthma patients in particular: Asthma is an illness associated with inflammation, and we wanted to determine whether the expected anti-inflammatory effects of the diet would affect the severity of their symptoms as they apparently had Marla's. Second, asthma symptoms are observable, vary from day to day, and are easy to monitor. And third, asthma had been linked to obesity even though weight loss alone had not been shown to improve symptoms.

Working with Warren Summer, chairman of the Pulmonary Medicine section at Louisiana State University Health Sciences Center, we designed a protocol for measuring asthma symptoms, and developed an eight-week study plan.

After establishing baseline values for asthma symptoms, weight, serum lipids, glucose, insulin, tumor necrosis factor-alpha and brain-derived neurotrophic factor (both indicators of inflammation), leptin and ketone levels, and levels of other chemicals, the study subjects were placed on a diet that—based on the average caloric requirement of 1,900 for men and 1,600 for women of normal weight—allowed the women to consume 320 calories and the men 380 calories (approximately 20 percent of normal) in the form of a canned meal-replacement shake on alternate days. On the days they weren't restricting, they were instructed to eat normally until they felt satisfied but not to intentionally overeat.

They were also given three questionnaires to fill out. The Asthma Symptom Utility Index Questionnaire, which is a tool for comparing the severity of symptoms among various individuals, was completed at the start of the study and every two weeks thereafter. Both the Asthma Quality of Life Questionnaire, in which patients assessed their perceived quality of life with relation to various issues, and the Asthma Control Questionnaire, which asked questions about the frequency and severity of various symptoms, were completed at the start and again at the end of the study.

THE QUESTION OF COMPLIANCE

Starting out, we were curious to know whether or not our study subjects would comply with the diet. In the end, we considered only one person a noncompleter because she admitted that she was eating on the down day, which meant we had achieved 90 percent compliance.

And apparently our subjects did not consider the regimen to be too onerous, because the self-assessed mood and energy levels of those who completed the study increased progressively during the first three weeks and remained elevated to the end.

They recorded their hunger levels every two hours while they were awake, and they did score hunger levels higher on the down day than on the up day. But the difference, on average, was only 0.4 on a scale of 1 to 10. And they were no hungrier on the up-days than they had been during the run up period when they recorded feelings of hunger in order for us to arrive at a baseline level. Nor did they report feeling hungrier as the study progressed. In fact, both overall hunger and the difference between up and down days declined over time. Their self-reports confirmed my own anecdotal impression that hunger on the down day was not so excessive as to prevent compliance.

Asthma Symptoms Improved Rapidly

One measurement of the severity of asthma symptoms is peak expiratory flow (PEF, or the amount of air a subject is able to blow out in a single breath). In our subjects the PEF showed a highly significant increase (more than 14 percent) beginning within three to four days of starting the diet, reached a peak at three weeks, and remained elevated for the duration (see chart). A second tool is to compare and measure the improvement in FEV1 (forced expiratory volume in one second) before and after administering a bronchodilator. This too was significantly improved by the end of the eight weeks.

Beyond these measurable results, however, our study participants showed highly significant improvement on the Asthma Symptom Utility Index, the Asthma Control Questionnaire, and

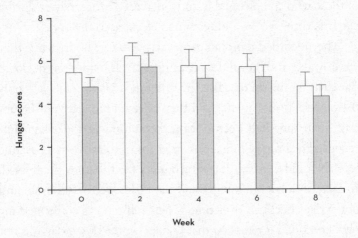

SELF-ASSESSED HUNGER DURING THE ASTHMA STUDY

White: average hunger score for the group on down days
Gray: average hunger score for the group on up days

PEAK EXPIRATORY FLOW

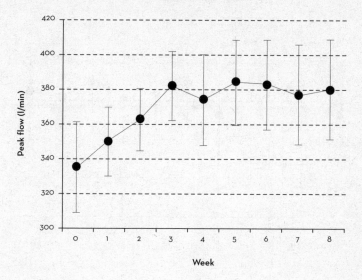

the Asthma Quality of Life Questionnaire starting within two weeks and lasting throughout the eight-week period. In fact, quality-of-life issues were significantly improved for all four indicators—asthma symptoms, activity limitations, emotional function, and environmental stimuli—at the end of the study as compared with those reported at the beginning. Improvement in mood and energy scores as recorded by the participants (see chart) was highly correlated with improvement in Peak Expiratory Flow.

There may have been a global mood improvement because the subjects were breathing better, but there also appears to be something about this diet that generates a euphoric or energized state of mind.

People following the Alternate-Day Diet universally experience an increase in energy after just a few down days. While

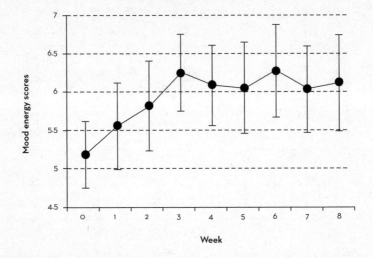

mood and energy also improved on the up days, there appears to be a greater change on the down days. Other studies of short-term fasting have shown an increase in circulating norepinephrine and cortisol levels. The improved mood may be mediated through an increase in the brain in the concentration of brain-derived neurotrophic factor, which acts to increase antidepressant action in the human brain and is known to increase in the brains of alternate-day-fed animals. Brain-derived neurotrophic factor is present in the peripheral bloodstream and actually is correlated with inflammation in the peripheral tissues, as opposed to the brain itself, where levels rise in response to alternate-day feeding.

By week 3 all the participants were in a "wired" state—they were talking more and were more energized—a change that is consistent with the increased brain function and activity levels found in studies restricting the calorie intake of both rodents and monkeys. Not only have these animals been shown to become more active, they have also become, in effect, "smarter."

Studies have shown that both calorie restriction and alternate-day feeding improve memory in rodents, and, as we have seen, alternate-day feeding has also been shown to improve resistance to experimental brain injury such as injection of a toxin into the hippocampus. This is important because the human brain is constantly being subjected to injury from metabolic insults and oxidative stress. So by extrapolation, the Alternate-Day Diet could also be expected to mitigate brain injury and preserve brain function.

REDUCTION IN OXIDATIVE STRESS

Elevated levels of nitrotyrosine in the blood is a research tool commonly used as an indicator of oxidative stress. It is elevated in people with heart disease and has been shown to be a hundred times more sensitive as an indicator of impending heart attack than the standard risk factors—cholesterol, blood pressure, and so on. The chart on the next page shows a 90 percent decline in nitrotyrosine levels over an eight-week period among participants in the Asthma Study. The samples were obtained fasting in the morning on two consecutive days after an up day (light-colored bars), and then after a down day (dark-colored bars) on study days 1 and 2, 15 and 16, 29 and 30, and 57 and 58. Note that:

- Most of the decline occurred by day 30.
- There is a significant reduction in nitrotyrosine after a single down day, especially comparing days 1 and 2, 15 and 16, and 29 and 30.
- Every subject had very low and very similar levels at the end of the study (very short standard error bars).

NITROTYROSINE LEVELS IN ASTHMA STUDY

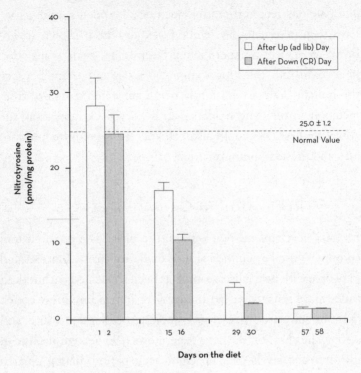

Source: Johnson et al., *Free Rad. Biol. Med.*

- The decline in nitrotyrosine level that occurs after a single down day (especially between days 1 and 2 and 15 and 16) means that these declines occurred without weight loss. If the subjects had eaten enough on the following up day to not lose weight, they still would have shown these declines. For this reason, we believe the alternate-day pattern works in the absence of weight loss.
- In contrast, in Mattson's study of subjects eating one meal a day there was no change in markers of oxidative stress

and inflammation.* The difference in the outcomes between these studies suggests that a period of about 36 hours is more effective than a period of 20 hours in activating the SIRT1-mediated CR mechanism.

The Anti-Inflammatory Effect

Oxidative damage and inflammation on the cellular level appear to be highly correlated in a complex cause-and-effect relationship. Oxidative damage is both a cause and a result of inflammation. But what exactly is inflammation? If you have a skin infection you'll see it manifested as redness, swelling, tenderness, and increased heat at the site of the infection. But these same changes can also occur in the walls of the arteries and, in the case of asthma, the lining of the small airways in the lung. The inflammation causes the lining to swell and the smooth muscle in the airways to narrow, which, in turn, causes wheezing and difficulty breathing. In fact, the main treatment for asthma is the use of an inhaled corticosteroid spray that suppresses the inflammation.

The alleviation of symptoms in patients in our Asthma Study would, in itself, have been an indication that they were experiencing a reduction in inflammation, but we also measured specific chemical substances in the bloodstream that are known to be indicators of inflammation. Over the course of the study, their levels of tumor necrosis factor-alpha, which is the most commonly used measure of inflammation, were reduced by two-thirds. Levels of TNF-alpha generally decline in association with weight loss, but the degree of reduction experienced by the

*Personal communication, Mark Mattson, 9-07.

people in our study was much greater than that reported in any study of weight loss we were able to find.

Brain-derived neurotrophic factor (BDNF), whose presence in peripheral circulation also indicates the presence of inflammation, declined 70 percent as well. We had to conclude from these results that the reduced energy supply (reduced calorie intake) on the down days was activating a powerful anti-inflammatory mechanism that increased progressively over a four-to-eight-week period.

In addition, levels of uric acid, a natural antioxidant, were increased, indicating an improvement in the body's antioxidant response. And levels of leptin—a pro-inflammatory substance that is, interestingly, also an indicator of hunger—decreased.

No other documented dietary or nondrug intervention has ever shown such a marked change in the levels of inflammation, meaning, we believe, that the Alternate-Day Diet has a potent effect on what is believed to be one of the main causes of a number of chronic and life-threatening illnesses, including arthritis and atherosclerosis.

OTHER SIGNIFICANT FINDINGS

Our study subjects did lose weight—about 8 percent of their initial body weight on average. Their levels of serum butyrate (an organic compound called a ketone) increased on down days, indicating compliance with the down-day dietary restriction and a shift in metabolism toward utilization of fatty acids—meaning that more fat was being used for energy instead of being stored.

A final positive finding was that their levels of HDL (good) cholesterol increased, creating a much more favorable ratio of good to bad (LDL) cholesterol, even though LDL levels them-

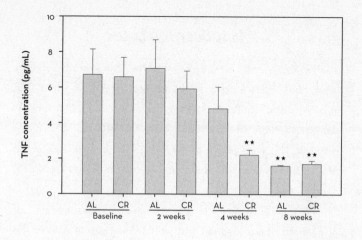

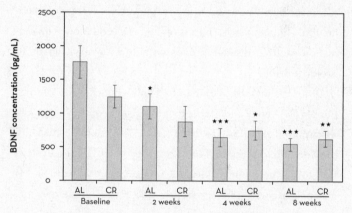

AL = ad lib, blood drawn the morning after an up day
CR = calories restricted to 20 percent, blood drawn
morning after a down day

selves did not decrease significantly. Their ratios of triglycerides to HDL also changed significantly, indicating a significant decrease in insulin resistance even though the reduction in insulin levels themselves did not reach statistical significance. This

Is It Ever Too Late?

Marla's experience as well as that of the Vallejo study subjects points out two related facts about calorie restriction: first, that it is never too late to start a program, and second, that there is an almost immediate onset of the positive effects that prolong survival. The average age of the Vallejo subjects at the start of the study was probably about seventy. Yet the diet clearly prolonged their lives.

We cannot measure long-term human survival because of the length of our lifespan, but we can measure effects of the Alternate-Day Diet on basic processes such as systemic inflammation. The premise is, therefore, that the reduction of inflammation reduces disease processes and, as a result, leads to prolonged life.

Prior to the Asthma Study, I had only a hunch, supported by people like Lenny and Marla, that the effects of the diet would be apparent within two to three weeks. The scientific literature provided no indication of how long it took for Calorie Restriction to act on a human disease process such as asthma. My colleagues and I were amazed to see that improvement occurred in the subjects' symptoms within three or four days.

More recently, the rapid onset of effect of Calorie Restriction on the longevity of fruit flies was demonstrated by Linda Partridge and her colleagues at University College, London. What the researchers found was that when fruit flies were put on a reduced-calorie diet, regardless of their ages, their longevity was increased within 48 hours. If they were then fed normally again, their death rate quickly returned to its original level.

finding alone suggests that the Alternate-Day eating pattern might be a way to treat prediabetics who don't require hypoglycemic agents or insulin.

WHAT IT ALL MEANS

The Asthma Study showed that symptoms were alleviated, pulmonary function was improved, and indicators of inflammation and oxidative stress declined as a result of the Alternate-Day Diet in this group of asthma sufferers. These findings, however, are consistent with the results in others who go on the Alternate-Day Diet, most of whom report feeling better within ten to fourteen days, with reduced symptoms of arthritis, allergies, and asthma, and other anecdotally observed improvements, within two weeks.

My colleagues and I believe—based on previous studies, on our own findings, and on personal anecdotal evidence—that the calorie restriction created by Alternate-Day dieting will have similar health benefits, in that it will reduce inflammation and oxidative damage while also helping to control body weight, for the general population. If, as we showed, the diet reduces the inflammation that is responsible for asthma symptoms, it is logical to assume that it will have a similar impact on all kinds of other chronic disorders, including heart disease. In other words, you too can lose weight, become more physically active, elevate your mood, become smarter, and, most important, increase your longevity by following the Alternate-Day Diet.

5.

SIRT1,
the "Rescue" Gene

Based on all the research and the study findings described so far, you should be convinced, as I am, of the efficacy of alternate-day dieting. You may, however, be wondering what it is about this plan that creates such benefits.

In large part, the answer appears to lie with a gene called SIRT1, which functions in mammals much the same way that a similar gene, Sir2, does in lower life forms such as yeast, worms, and fruit flies. Our bodies are made up of many different kinds of genes that perform myriad different functions. Some are responsible for determining eye, hair, and skin color, others may put us more or less at risk for particular diseases, and some work by activating or deactivating other genes. Sir2 and SIRT1 fall into this last category. These and other, similar genes are called "silent information regulators" because they appear to sense the levels of particular substances in the body and turn on downstream chemical reactions that regulate the manner in which we respond to these substances on a cellular level.

In 1999, researchers working in the lab of Leonard Guarente

at MIT reported that brewer's yeast lived longer when it contained higher levels of a gene called Sir2. With input from other researchers, it was established that reducing the food supply (instituting calorie restriction) to the yeast prolonged its lifespan through activation of Sir2. Since then, it has been demonstrated that the equivalent gene (called SIRT1) is activated in calorie-restricted mammals, including rats, mice, and humans.

Many researchers are now investigating the complex nature of SIRT1 and how it affects our bodies—particularly how it is activated and how it conveys resistance to stress—and new information is constantly forthcoming. The interesting question is why Sir2 and SIRT1 exist. Because these genes are found in the most ancient life forms and appear to be present in all species in various forms, the typical speculation is that they act to protect the organism in times of adversity, such as when there is an inadequate food supply, allowing the animal to survive until food conditions improve. Whatever the original purpose of these genes, however, the recent scientific discoveries that have allowed us to understand (and eventually control) how they act are nothing short of miraculous. Among the most prominent of the scientists investigating these mechanisms is David Sinclair at the Harvard Medical School.

SIRT1 TO THE RESCUE

When a cell is exposed to fatal stress, such as extreme heat or starvation, it reacts one of two ways: It either necroses and dies immediately or it begins a process called apoptosis, which leads to a slower but inevitable programmed cell death.

Sinclair and his colleagues have shown that SIRT1 prevents this cell suicide by interfering with the action of a protein called

What Exactly Is a "Stress Response"?

The most widely accepted theory of why calorie restriction prevents disease and/or delays the onset of age-related diseases is called "hormesis," which means that a harmful stress—one that might be fatal in large quantities—is beneficial in small amounts. Thus, if an animal is starved, it dies, but if its daily calorie intake is reduced to 60 percent of normal, it lives longer in very good health. (If calories are reduced to less than 60 percent, the average lifespan is shortened.) The physiologic events that occur in response to a nonfatal stimulus constitute the stress response. At the level of gene expression, the stress response is believed to be initiated by SIRT1 activation. The downstream effects of SIRT1 activation include reduced oxidative stress and inflammation and reduced fat storage and anti-apoptosis.

In humans, as in animals, the stress response is probably "dose-related." That is, zero calorie intake every other day activates the mechanism more intensely than daily calorie restriction. But, as I've said, and as Eric Ravussin also determined in his three-week study of volunteers who were employees in his lab (see page 40), most humans would not willingly adhere to an every-other-day eating pattern on a long-term basis. That said, the Alternate-Day Diet will activate the stress response to the metabolic and oxidative insults to which we are constantly subjected.

BAX, which initiates the apoptosis process. This gives the cell time to repair the damage done by the stressor and continue to function normally.

SIRT1 is "turned on" to do its work in the body through a shift in the relative levels of the coenzymes nicotinamide and NAD+. When NAD+ is present, SIRT1 is activated. When, through a biochemical reaction, NAD+ is turned into nicotinamide (which is NAD+ minus one electron), SIRT1 is inhibited.

ALTERNATE-DAY TURNS ON SIRT1

You may be wondering what all this has to do with the Alternate-Day Diet. On the simplest level, the answer is that when energy (i.e., serum glucose) supplied to the cell is as low as it is in calorie restriction, the level of NAD+ rises, turning on SIRT1. David Sinclair has described the series of events that occur on the cellular level in response to reduced calorie intake as a metaphor for making a 911 call in an emergency. SIRT1 answers the call and dispatches the "rescuers" that prevent the stressed cells from dying. Some organs, such as the liver, are capable of regenerating themselves after cells are lost, but others, most notably the heart and the brain, are not. Preventing loss of critical cells due to apoptosis in organs that do not regenerate may, therefore, be one way SIRT1 promotes longevity.

Anthony E. Civitarese, Eric Ravussin, and their colleagues published a study that looked at three groups of overweight but not obese people for a period of six months. A control group ate 100 percent of their calorie requirements daily; a second group received 25 percent less; and a third group had their calorie intake reduced by 12.5 percent while also increasing their calorie expenditure through exercise by 12.5 percent. After six months,

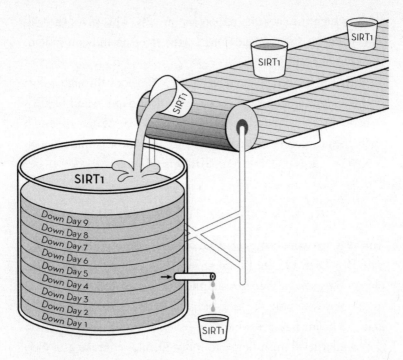

A single 36-hour period of low-energy supply (reduced calories) causes a rise in levels of the SIRT1 protein that diminishes over several days. Each down day causes a similar rise in SIRT1, and levels remain elevated even when eating normally every other day.

the researchers found, by doing biopsies of the subjects' thigh muscle, that both those who were restricted 25 percent and those who combined exercise with a 12.5 percent calorie restriction had more mitochondria and less free-radical damage to their DNA, and had activated SIRT1. These results confirmed those of a previous study by the same team that showed SIRT1 activation after three weeks of eating every other day. Based on their findings, the researchers stated that eating fewer calories "can improve whole body metabolism in conjunction with an increase in SIRT1 gene expression in skeletal muscle. These results raise the possibility that SIRT1 may contribute to more efficient metabolism, less oxidative stress, and increased longevity in humans as it does in lower organisms."

Genes are "expressed" in response to a variety of stimuli. In the Ravussin study, SIRT1 was expressed over the six-month duration of the study. But it probably only takes skipping a meal to increase our SIRT1 levels. In mice it has been shown that a 24-hour fast activates SIRT1 and that the increased activity is still measurable more than 24 hours after the end of the fast. This effect is not unlike that which my colleagues and I have observed in asthmatics. Not only were their markers for oxidative stress reduced after only one down day, indicating the rapid onset of SIRT1, but after following the Alternate-Day Diet for several weeks and then stopping, their symptoms remained improved for approximately ten to fourteen days, suggesting that SIRT1 was still active and its downstream effects were still operating. Formation of SIRT1 protein and its *gradual* decay over a period of days would explain this phenomenon.

Furthermore, based on our findings, we believe that alternate-day calorie restriction without actual fasting as provided by alternate-day dieting is sufficient to create the stress reaction that activates SIRT1 and also that its expression will continue to intensify and strengthen as long as this eating pattern is continued.

It is highly likely, therefore, that this ancient genetic mechanism functions in humans much the same way it does in mice.

SIRT1, NF-Kappa B, and Inflammation

Another effect of SIRT1 is to inhibit a protein called NF-kappa B, which causes inflammation. Inflammation exists to defend against germs and tumors, but it can also act in a harmful way to cause cancer, arthritis, asthma, heart disease, and neurodegeneration. What this means is that activation of SIRT1 could be expected to reduce the incidence of these diseases caused by inflammation.

SIRT1 Can Also Make You Thin

SIRT1 has a broad range of effects on metabolism. For example, limiting food intake increases SIRT1 activity in fat cells, causing fat to move into the bloodstream, where it is used as energy.

In the same way that SIRT1 acts upon BAX to prevent cellular apoptosis, it also works to inhibit fat storage by turning off another gene, called PPAR-gamma. Because PPAR-gamma is responsible for allowing the deposition of fat, fat storage is inhibited when it is deactivated.

In terms of weight loss this is good news not only because, obviously, the more fat you store the fatter you become, but also because reduced levels of body fat mean an increased ratio of muscle to fat. Also, because there are far more mitochondria in muscle tissue, it burns calories more efficiently than fat. More muscle means faster metabolism, which means that you will use the calories you eat more quickly.

In terms of health and increased longevity, however, the effect of SIRT1 on fat storage may have even greater significance because chemicals called inflammatory cytokines (such as tumor necrosis factor-alpha, previously discussed), which cause the chronic inflammation that contributes to the accumulation of damage to the organs we describe as aging, are produced by fat cells. What this means is that activating SIRT1 in fat cells could significantly slow the aging process and prevent specific diseases such as Type 2 diabetes, atherosclerosis, arthritis, osteoporosis, neurodegenerative disorders such as Alzheimer's disease, and some types of cancer, which are very probably mediated by pro-inflammatory cytokines.

As Dr. Guarente has said, "The accumulation of WAT [white adipose tissue—i.e., fat] during ageing is associated with several adverse complications, such as insulin resistance, Type 2 diabetes and atherosclerosis. Given the impact of SIRT1 on PPAR-g activity and because PPAR-g activity helps determine age-related insulin resistance, SIRT1 may have an important role in metabolic diseases and link the effects of food consumption to body fat mass and diseases of ageing."

Boosting Your Levels of SIRT1

Based on the many apparent benefits of activating SIRT1, it would seem logical to make sure it's working for you as much as possible. With the discovery that high levels of NAD+ activated SIRT1, the possibility that naturally occurring chemicals might "artificially" turn on this mechanism occurred to David Sinclair and workers at Biomol Laboratories. Testing a "library" of thousands of compounds, they found that a chemical named resveratrol and sixteen other plant-derived substances prolonged the lifespan of yeast by up to 70 percent.

An antioxidant known to be present in red wine, resveratrol had been targeted by Serge Renaud in the early 1990s as possibly responsible for what he termed the "French Paradox." He suggested that drinking red wine might be a factor in the explanation of why the French, despite eating a diet high in saturated fat and cholesterol as compared with Americans, had a much lower risk of heart disease. In other words, drinking red wine might have been protecting them against heart disease.

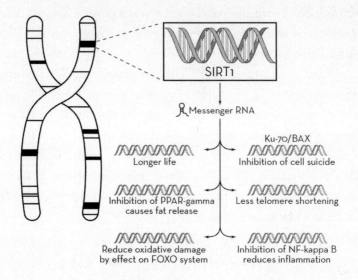

According to the article "Therapeutic Potential of Resveratrol: The *in vivo* Evidence," by David Sinclair and Joseph A. Baur, published in *Nature Reviews* (June 2006), "Since then, dozens of reports have shown that resveratrol can prevent or slow the progression of a wide variety of illnesses, including cancer, cardiovascular disease and ischaemic injuries [i.e., stroke], as well as enhance stress resistance and extend the lifespans of various organisms from yeast to vertebrates."

The article cites numerous studies in which resveratrol has been shown to inhibit tumor growth in rodents, to reduce the markers of oxidative stress in hypertensive rats, to reduce inflammation, and to reduce brain damage following a stroke. In fact, Sinclair and Baur conclude, "It is becoming clear that resveratrol and more potent mimetics show great promise in the treatment of the leading causes of morbidity and mortality in the Western

Alcohol: A Little Is Good

Drinking alcohol in moderation, up to two drinks per day for men and one drink a day for women, reduces heart attacks by 30 to 40 percent compared with nondrinkers. In people under age forty, however, there is no health benefit, since heart attack is rare in any case. Drinking it all on one or two days of the week doesn't do it. And the kind of alcohol doesn't matter. Red wine is probably no better.

The incidence of breast cancer in women and colon cancer in both men and women is higher among those who are moderate drinkers than among non-drinkers. If you do drink, taking a folic acid supplement appears to reduce the cancer risk.

In addition to being potentially addictive and causing a third of all traffic fatalities, excess drinking increases the risk of a variety of cancers as well as high blood pressure and liver disease. Moreover, you can get the same heart health benefit from increasing your exercise level, so don't feel compelled to start drinking if you don't already.

world. . . . Could resveratrol and similar molecules form the next class of wonder-drugs? Clinical trials are currently underway in several locations . . . and could soon answer this question."

Although there is still much to be learned about exactly what mechanisms are responsible for these effects, it seems clear that at least one of the ways resveratrol works is to activate SIRT1.

If Resveratrol Can Turn on SIRT1, Why Not Just Skip the Diet?

Wouldn't it be great if we could forget dieting altogether and just pop a couple of resveratrol capsules along with our daily vitamins? Whether or not this might be a viable alternative probably depends on whether you are trying to get the potential health benefits of resveratrol or to lose weight. There is a big range in possible doses, but resveratrol and related chemicals may well have weight-loss effects in addition to significant health benefits.

Two landmark studies that appeared toward the end of 2006 showed for the first time that resveratrol had effects in mice similar to those seen in lower animals. In the first, David Sinclair, Rafael de Cabo, and associates showed that mice fed a

Does Fat Make You Dumb?

Another negative aspect of obesity that is not widely appreciated is the very significant effect it has on mental ability. Numerous studies document the fact that obesity and high-saturated-fat, high-calorie diets negatively affect cognitive function in animals and humans. Insulin resistance and Type 2 diabetes magnify this effect. Resveratrol has been shown to improve neuromuscular function in mice, indicating a positive effect on the central nervous system.

In addition, resveratrol has been shown to reverse severe cognitive deficits in an Alzheimer's disease mouse model. This is the first potential agent that could actually improve cognitive function in neurodegenerative diseases such as Alzheimer's.

high-calorie diet and 24 milligrams per kilogram of body weight of resveratrol survived 31 percent longer than mice fed a standard diet. Another group of mice fed 5 mg per kg of body weight showed many of the same health benefits as the higher dose. Among other findings, the resveratrol-fed mice did not develop atherosclerosis, had improved motor function, and showed an increased number of mitochondria, all in the absence of weight loss. The improved motor function in this study is an indication that the negative effects of a high-calorie diet on the brain were reversed by the resveratrol.

The second study appeared in the journal *Cell* in December 2006. Here, scientists working with David Sinclair and Johan Auwerx in Illkirch, France, showed that mice fed 200 to 400 mg of resveratrol per kg of body weight mixed with their food became lean and were able to run twice as far. It is possible, then, that humans could lose weight if they were willing to take 15 or 20 grams of resveratrol per day. But this dose is extremely high, and its safety has not been established at that level.

The resveratrol-fed mice had much bigger and more numerous mitochondria in their muscle cells, and the authors concluded this was a direct effect of the resveratrol. In addition, the animals fed resveratrol had faster metabolisms (greater energy expenditure) and improved results on tests of the central nervous system, such as balance and strength. They also had less insulin resistance and improved glucose tolerance, both of which are abnormal in many overweight people.

Dysfunction of the mitochondria is seen in heart disease, neurodegenerative diseases (like Alzheimer's), and metabolic diseases (like Type 2 diabetes), all of which could potentially be treated with resveratrol-type drugs. Also, both exercise and calorie reduction increase the number and function of the mitochondria

Resveratrol Supplements and Drugs

At the moment, resveratrol is being sold by many vendors on the Internet, and it is possible that the Alternate-Day Diet might be even more effective if you were also to take resveratrol, but an effective dose would probably have to be quite high, and the risks of taking high doses over the long term have not yet been established.

David Sinclair, in partnership with Christoph Westphal, has formed a corporation, Sirtris, to develop drugs based on resveratrol as well as other SIRT1 activators. Reportedly, pharmaceutical giants such as Merck and Pfizer are also interested in developing SIRT1 activators.

and are the cornerstones of treatment of metabolic syndrome, a condition involving multiple risk factors for cardiovascular disease, including abdominal obesity, insulin resistance and glucose intolerance, elevated blood pressure, and a pro-inflammatory state. Thus SIRT1 activators like resveratrol might be very useful for treating this common condition.

Resveratrol was effective in reversing the cognitive loss in a mouse model of Alzheimer's disease and in preventing the death of neurons associated with the process. This lends promise to the possibility of effective treatment of Alzheimer's disease.

Part Two

THE ALTERNATE-DAY
DIET PROGRAM

6.

Starting the Alternate-Day Diet

Given everything we know about human biology and psychology—particularly about our deeply ingrained drive to eat when the eating is good and to turn to food in times of emotional stress—it makes sense to be as prepared as possible before you begin this or any other diet program. Remember that the primitive, reptilian part of your brain is going to be telling you to eat, eat, eat! So you need to use the higher, thinking brain you've been given as a human to counteract and control that primitive urge—you need to be educated. Following are a few simple things you should know and do before you begin.

DETERMINE YOUR CALORIE NEEDS

On the down days of the Alternate-Day Diet, you will start by eating approximately 20 percent of the calories you require to maintain your weight. What that means, of course, is that you need to determine how many calories you're consuming right now.

There are a number of ways you can do that. If, for example, your weight has been steady over a period of time, you could keep a food diary to help you figure out how many calories you've been taking in on a daily basis. The trouble with this method, however, is that it requires you to know exactly how many calories are in the food you eat and to be extremely vigilant and completely honest with yourself. Most people just can't or won't do that.

You may not mean to cheat, but chances are you're not going to stop and make a note each time you "have a little taste" of something or eat a couple of chips out of someone else's bag or a couple of fries off your dinner companion's plate. And having to figure out the calorie content of everything you put in your mouth can be daunting, if not impossible. Maybe your broccoli was sautéed in a little bit of oil—but how much? And exactly how much broccoli are you actually eating? These days many of us eat many of our meals outside the home. If you're in a restaurant, will you have a food scale with you? Will you take the broccoli off your plate and put it on the scale before you eat it? Surely you can see how easy it is to eat more (or less) than you think you are. So how do you avoid the inaccuracies that come with this kind of portion distortion?

Determine Your RMR

One way to determine how many calories you *need* to maintain your weight is to figure out your resting metabolic rate (RMR), which is similar to your basal metabolic rate (BMR). Your RMR is a measure of how many calories you burn just by staying alive. In fact, the energy (that is, calories) required to perform your bodily functions—breathing, pumping blood throughout your body, and maintaining your body temperature, for example—can account for up to 70 percent of your total calorie intake.

The most accurate way to determine your RMR is through a series of tests that require specialized equipment to which most of us do not have access. Several mathematical formulas have been developed to estimate RMR, however. The one that is generally accepted as the "gold standard" is called the Harris-Benedict equation. It requires a bit of simple arithmetic (or you can use an automatic calculator found online at several websites). Here's the equation.

HARRIS-BENEDICT EQUATION

RMR for Men = 66 + (6.23 × weight in pounds) + (12.7 × height in inches) – (6.8 × age)
RMR for Women = 655 + (4.35 × weight in pounds) + (4.7 × height in inches) – (4.7 × age)

For example:

A 30-year-old man who weighs 150 pounds and is 6 feet tall would figure his RMR this way: 66 + 934.50 + 914.4 – 204 = 1,710.90

A 30-year-old woman who weighs 125 pounds and is 5 feet, 6 inches tall would figure her RMR this way: 655 + 543.75 + 305.5 – 141 = 1,363.25

THE HARRIS-BENEDICT MARGIN OF ERROR

Because of multiple factors, including the ratio of fat to muscle and variations in metabolic rate from one individual to another, there is a standard deviation of 14 percent above and below the number of calories determined by the Harris-Benedict equation.

The Activity Factor

The Harris-Benedict formula requires that you factor your activity level into your daily calorie allotment. Harris-Benedict figures activity levels this way:

Sedentary (little or no exercise, you work at a desk job): RMR x 1.2

Lightly active (light exercise or sports 1 to 3 days a week): RMR x 1.375

Moderately active (moderate exercise or sports 3 to 5 days a week): RMR x 1.55

Very active (hard exercise or sports 6 to 7 days a week): RMR x 1.725

Extra active (hard exercise or sports daily, working at a physical job, or training for a marathon or other competitive sport twice a day): RMR x 1.9

Note: To avoid having to do the calculations above, you can use the online Calorie Calculator tool at johnsonupdaydown daydiet.com/how-to-do-the-diet.html to estimate your normal calorie requirements and your down-day calories.

But with all due respect to Harris-Benedict, I've found that just as there's a problem letting people figure out how many calories they consume in a day, there's also a problem with allowing people to determine their own activity level. Just as most of us underestimate how much we eat, we also tend to overestimate our level of activity. In fact, if you're overweight, you're probably doing both right now. A study published in the *New England Journal of Medicine* in 1992 indicates that people who are trying to lose weight (and most overweight people are perpetually trying to lose weight) may underestimate the amount they're eating by as much as 47 percent and overestimate their activity levels by 51 percent. I'm not saying this to make you feel bad; it's just a fact of human nature, and one of which I've been as guilty as the next guy.

It's not unusual to hear a woman who is five-foot-five and weighs 200 pounds say that she does vigorous aerobic activity 60 to 90 minutes six days a week and "hardly eats anything." While this is probably not impossible, it seems unlikely. So to help counteract this natural tendency, I recommend that you calculate your RMR using the activity level that is *one below* the level you *think* applies to you. Activity level can have a significant effect on our daily caloric needs. If you exercise very little or not at all, exercise little, or are sedentary (no exercise), the activity factor multiplier is 1.2, which I have found is probably the best factor for most people. Of course, there will be the rare case of a mountain climber doing a traverse of Mount McKinley in February who is burning 8,000 to 10,000 calories per day and for whom a high activity multiplier is justified—but that's clearly the exception rather than the rule.

As a "real life" guideline the National Weight Control Registry, which studies people who have lost weight and maintained long-term weight loss, has shown that the men eat 1,700 calories and the women 1,400 per day, and that on average they burned 400 calories a day in aerobic exercise.

This means that if the equation estimate is 2,000 calories, there is a 95 percent chance the actual number you require may be anywhere from 1,440 to 2,560. The good news, however, is that if you are calculating your down-day requirement, 20 percent of the calories you require could be anywhere from 288 to 512. The average of these figures would be 400 calories, which is a good enough estimate. Consuming 100 calories more or less on your down day will not change your results.

The Value of Self-Monitoring

Keep a Journal

I strongly recommend that during the first two to three weeks on the Alternate-Day Diet, you use a commercially prepared canned shake or bar on the down day to make sure that your calorie intake is no more than 20 percent of normal. Everyone appears to lose weight if they adhere to this level on the down day. At around three weeks, however, you may find your weight loss is slowing. This may be because you are unconsciously increasing your calorie intake. At this point it is, therefore, important to begin monitoring your eating.

Based on everything you've read so far, it should be quite obvious that our appetites exceed our caloric requirements. Or, as I've said, our appetite-control mechanism is broken. As a result, if we want to lose or maintain a healthy body weight, we have to employ external measures of how much we are eating. We do this commonly by getting on the scale. Another method of self-monitoring is to keep a food log. Many studies have shown food logs to be effective for weight loss and weight-loss maintenance. Recording what, when, how much, and why we eat produces both immediate and delayed feedback by keeping us consciously aware of what we are eating and, later, what we ate.

Seeing what you're putting in your mouth written down in black and white right before your eyes makes it harder to fool yourself. And knowing that you have to write it down may also make you think twice before you eat when you're really not hungry. How often have you had the classic self-delusional experience of planning to eat one potato chip and discovering half an hour later that the bag is empty? Would it have happened if you had written down each potato chip? Of course not. Writing down each chip you eat may sound ridiculous, but it works. There are other good reasons for keeping a journal as well.

If you weigh yourself (as you should) before you begin the Alternate-Day Diet and write the number down in your journal, you'll always remember where you started from. Then, as you continue to weigh yourself at regular intervals, you'll see how much progress you've made. Nothing succeeds like success. And there's no better way to keep yourself motivated than to see how much progress you're making. If you see, written in black and white, that you have lost weight, you will feel better and you will be more likely to stick with the plan.

There is one caveat, however. Don't weigh yourself every day, because your weight will fluctuate considerably between up and down days. Always weigh yourself on the morning after a down day and preferably at 6-day or 8-day intervals, because doing that will give you the most accurate picture of your true progress. And you don't want to make yourself feel bad by weighing after an up day.

A third reason to keep a journal is to track the improvement of any health issues you might have when you begin the diet. I strongly suggest that you have your fasting cholesterol, insulin, and glucose levels checked at the outset—particularly if you already know that any or all of them are elevated.

If you have asthma, you should use a peak flow meter to record baseline levels of peak expiratory flow and if possible have pulmonary function studies (FEV1) done. Then monitor the changes in these levels at regular intervals. If you have arthritis, record the range of motion in your affected joints and the amount of soreness you are experiencing.

The various conditions for which my colleagues and I have seen improvement in people on the Alternate-Day Diet include insulin resistance, asthma, seasonal allergies, autoimmune disease (rheumatoid arthritis), osteoarthritis, inflammatory central nervous system lesions (Tourette's syndrome, Ménière's disease), cardiac arrhythmias (frequent extrasystoles, atrial fibrillation), menopause-related hot flashes, and infectious diseases of viral, bacterial, and fungal origin (toenail fungus, periodontal disease, viral URIs).

And, finally, keep track of your quality-of-life issues, as my colleagues and I did with the patients in our Asthma Study. Are the symptoms of whatever health issue you have improving? Are you able to do more on a daily basis than you did before beginning the diet? Do you feel that you have more energy? Are you in a better state mentally and emotionally than you were starting out? Once you see how much progress you're making, you'll have the positive reinforcement that will help you stick with the program.

The key to compliance with any kind of diet or health plan is to self-monitor. I learned this many years ago at the University of Michigan when I was working with Edwin Thomas at the School of Social Work to treat a man with Tourette's syndrome, an illness whose symptoms consist of involuntary tics and vocalizations. We gave him a small counting device and instructed him to click it every time he became aware of a tic or of making an involuntary sound. After just two days, the incidence of his tic

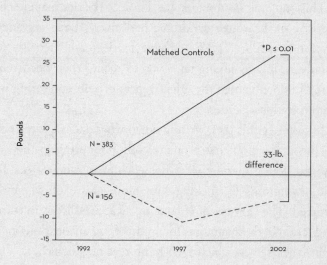

WEIGHT LOSS OVER 10 YEARS
Case-Controlled Comparison
in Separate Communities after Blackburn

Matched Controls

*P ≤ 0.01

Pounds

N = 383

33-lb.
difference

N = 156

1992   1997   2002

One of the few long-term weight-loss studies available was done by Dr. George Blackburn at Harvard Medical School, in which participants consumed either a meal-replacement shake or bar for one or two meals each day for ten years. Compared to a control group who ate normally, there was an average 33-pound difference in weight. The diet group lost 7 pounds and the control group gained 26 pounds. This study is important because it demonstrates (1) that people who eat without restriction are going to gain weight over time if they do not control their intake; (2) that daily self-monitoring works; and (3) that meal-replacement products are effective aids to facilitate self-monitoring.

was decreased to one ten-thousandth of frequency before treatment began, and remained at that lower level for the duration of our study.

This outcome was remarkable, because the tics that are characteristic of Tourette's syndrome had always been considered completely involuntary. Being able to decrease them so profoundly, simply by taking an action to record their occurrence, therefore documented the effectiveness of self-monitoring with relation to this disorder.

In terms of this diet, writing down what one is experiencing is a physical action that promotes self-monitoring in the same way that young man's clicker helped him to monitor his Tourette's symptoms by making him more aware of when they occurred. The very act of enhancing awareness leads in turn to a reduction of the symptoms (or, in this case, unconscious eating habits) themselves, which then reinforces new behaviors. Once you become aware that something is working because you have concrete, written proof of your progress, you will be that much more likely to continue what you've been doing.

How Much Are You Really Eating?

In addition to keeping a journal, there are other simple tools you can use to become more aware of your consumption.

- ***Learn to read a food label.***
  Food labels tell you not only how much is in a package but also how many portions the package contains. Many of us suffer from what I like to call "container eating," which means that we tend to consume whatever the package contains. This can be as many as four or more por-

tions, and the calorie count on the package is for only one of those portions. Reading the label will help you to become more aware not only of what a single portion *should be* but also of how many calories you're *actually consuming.*

- **Use measuring tools to control your consumption.** Measuring spoons, liquid and dry measuring cups, and small food scales are inexpensive and readily available. Buy them if you don't already own them, and use them to keep yourself honest. Many diet books will tell you that a "portion" of meat is the size of a deck of cards or that a tablespoon of butter is the length from the tip of your thumb to the first joint. But I find that these approximations are often an excuse for overindulging. Not only is using calibrated measuring implements a much more accurate way to self-monitor but also the simple act of measuring will make you much more aware of what a proper portion actually is.

KEEP YOURSELF HYDRATED

More and more people these days are walking around with water bottles in their purse, briefcase, or backpack—maybe you're one of them. But did you know that some studies indicate that up to 75 percent of Americans still suffer from some degree of dehydration every day?

The specific amount of water you need to remain appropriately hydrated depends on many factors, including your health, your activity level, and where you live. On average, you lose two quarts a day through your sweat, breath, urine, and stool. When you perspire you lose more, up to a quart per hour when you exercise vigorously.

Even minor dehydration can make you feel out of sorts, headachy, and lightheaded. You may feel fatigued and find it difficult to think clearly. *Chronic* mild dehydration can lead to kidney stones and even bladder cancer.

Getting enough fluid means that you have to drink throughout the day. If you drink a cup of liquid between meals and a cup or more with each meal, you should stay pretty well hydrated. One easy solution is to keep a one-quart container with you during the day and drink it between meals.

You can't just wait until you're thirsty, because by then you're already somewhat dehydrated. Older people in particular can become dehydrated because they often don't realize they're thirsty. Beyond that, we often think we're hungry when we're really thirsty and might decide to eat when we should really be drinking. When you feel hungry, your first response should be to drink a glass of water.

The *type* of liquid you consume is also important in terms of weight control because of the sugar and empty calories so many drinks contain. Nondiet soda, which is full of sugar and, therefore, empty calories, makes up one-quarter of all the liquids Americans drink! If you are serious about long-term weight control, make it a habit *never to drink sodas that contain sugar.* They have been implicated as primarily responsible for the rise in obesity among children and diabetes among women. Diet sodas, however, are fine in moderation. There is no good scientific evidence to support the purported negative side effects from use of artificial sweeteners such as saccharin, aspartame, and sucralose, but the long-term high-volume use of such products by children has not been studied yet.

YOUR ALTERNATE-DAY DIET JOURNAL

DATE	TIME	FOOD & AMOUNT	CALORIES	HUNGER LEVEL 1-10	MOOD LEVEL 1-10
1/1	9 AM	Oatmeal, 1 cup	175	5	7

Create a journal along the lines of the sample above. Recording what, when, and how much you eat will automatically reduce your intake and mindless eating. It is important to enter the food and amount immediately after eating. At a minimum record what you ate and the estimated calories. If you consume more than you planned, write it down anyway. Cheating doesn't help you. But noting your hunger and food levels, on a rough scale of 1 to 10, will reveal patterns of emotional eating. The more detail you write down, the more effective the program will be for you. Adapt the journal to suit your personal needs.

Coffee, Tea, and Caffeine

Coffee has long been blamed for a variety of ills, but more recently it has been shown to be a very safe beverage. Drinking up to six cups of coffee a day reduces the risk of kidney stones, gallstones, and Type 2 diabetes, and, as a bonus, suicide rates are 70 percent lower among coffee drinkers than non-coffee drinkers. One commonly held myth is that caffeine causes dehydration. In fact, up to six cups of coffee per day does not increase diuresis (water loss through the kidneys) any more than plain water.

So caffeine-containing beverages can make up at least part of your daily fluid requirement. When you follow the Alternate-Day Diet, however, you may find that your energy level is very high and that you have trouble falling asleep. For this reason you may want to limit your consumption of caffeine, especially later in the day.

Tea has enjoyed a recent upswing in popularity because of the putative benefits of the polyphenols it contains, especially EGCG (epigallocatechin gallate). Tea may reduce the incidence of cancer and heart disease, but the evidence to support this is to date not convincing.

Black tea is made with leaves that have been fermented, whereas green tea is made with unfermented leaves. Both types contain caffeine and have the same benefits as coffee, including a mild antidepressant effect and a reduction in the risk of kidney and gallstones.

One of the most effective ways to reduce calories is to drink sparkling water, perhaps with a squeeze of lemon juice or lime juice or an ounce of fruit juice added.

Also, you may be surprised to know that—contrary to what the dairy industry would have you believe—there is no good health reason to drink milk. Dairy fat is saturated, which means that it promotes atherosclerosis and adds superfluous calories, and there are many safer and easier ways to obtain additional calcium if necessary. (For more on this, see Chapter 7.)

Finally, many plant-based foods also contain a lot of water. Think of lettuce, tomatoes, cucumbers, zucchini, melons, and peaches, for example. Interestingly, these are also foods that are generally low in calories. And as I've already said, there is evidence that eating foods with a high water content, which means that they have fewer calories with relation to volume, is also an effective way to reduce overall calorie consumption.

As with calories, the most important factor is awareness during the day of the need to maintain hydration. There are a thousand appealing varieties of bottled water available. Buy a case or two and put the bottles where you will drink them during the course of the day—in the refrigerator, at your desk, in your car, and so forth.

Get Yourself Moving

Exercise protects against

- heart disease
- high blood pressure
- high cholesterol
- cancer, especially of the colon and breast

- adult-onset Type 2 diabetes
- arthritis
- osteoporosis
- constipation
- depression
- weight gain

Exercise also builds muscle, which is a critical component of weight control. The more muscle you have, the more energy your body uses, the more calories you burn. As we age or if we are inactive, there is a shift in body composition from muscle to fat. The way to counteract that shift is through exercise, and it is never too late to begin. Studies show that elderly people gain great benefits from exercise programs.

The best way to build muscle is through strength training, also called resistance training, which generally requires some kind of equipment. The equipment can be as simple as handheld weights or elastic bands, or as complex as the machines found in professional gyms. It is based on working specific muscles or muscle groups to "failure" (the point at which you can't do another repetition) in order to increase their mass and strength.

In addition to strength or resistance training, it's also important to do aerobic exercise, which improves heart function by increasing its pumping efficiency.

Cardio Versus Strength Training— Finding the Balance

The American College of Sports Medicine recommends that you do strength training no more than three times a week to give your body the time to repair the microscopic muscle tears this kind of training creates, but also states that you can do cardio-vascular exercise every day. I would add that you *should* do cardio exercise at least five times a week. A standard recommendation for an effective but not overstrenuous exercise program with which I agree is 30 minutes of cardio five times a week (doing more will further decrease your risk of heart disease) plus a minimum of 30 minutes of strength training three days a week, with a day off between each session.

I'm not going to recommend or illustrate specific strength-training exercises here because there are many books by professional trainers that do just that. What I do suggest is that you consult a good trainer at a local gym to determine how much exercise of what type you should be doing, depending on your health and your normal level of activity. It's easier, in any case, to do strength training at a gym, with a buddy, or with a trainer. If you have to be somewhere because you've made an appointment, you're more likely to do it, and working with a professional will ensure that you're doing the exercises correctly so that they produce the best results and you don't inadvertently injure yourself.

The key to successful strength training is, as I've said, to attempt to work a particular muscle or group of muscles to the point of exhaustion—called muscle failure. The problem is that many people, especially women, don't like the feeling of muscle exhaustion and therefore don't try hard enough to get the maximum stimulation, which is what causes the muscle to grow.

Each muscle group in the body needs to be trained. Usually these groups are broken into legs, chest, back, arms, and shoulders, with one or two groups worked on different days. Here's my own routine to use as an example:

Monday: legs (leg press, squats, leg curl, and calf raise)
Wednesday: chest and back (lat pull down, seated row, shrugs, bench press, flies, and inclined bench press)
Friday: arms and shoulders (overhead press, front and lateral straight-arm dumbbell raises, curl and triceps cable pushdown)

In 45 minutes I do four sets of 15 repetitions for most of these exercises. Overall, I enjoy the process more than I enjoy aerobic exercise. I like the social activity of going to the gym and the challenge of doing my personal best. In fact, I find that there is something inherently physically satisfying about lifting weights.

Whether aerobic or strength training is more valuable for health is unclear. Strength training increases muscle mass and is essential for counteracting the natural age-related loss of muscle and increase in body fat with which we all contend. Studies show that even as little as 10 to 15 minutes of resistance exercise for each muscle group (1 to 2 minutes per group) three times a week is effective for maintaining muscle mass. Of course, more is better, and anyone can do it.

The simplest form of aerobic or cardiovascular activity is walking, which confers many of the same benefits of more vigorous activity. Almost anyone can walk, and even in bad weather there's usually someplace you *can* walk. In some places, for example, there are groups that meet regularly to walk in a local indoor mall. Again, it would be best to hook up with a buddy with whom you can walk. If you're walking with a friend, it will go that much more quickly. As you gain strength and energy (and you *will*), you can begin to alternate running and walking—run for a few minutes, then walk a few minutes, then run again.

After a while you might even give up walking altogether for running!

Also, if you enjoy a particular sport, you can satisfy your cardiovascular exercise that way—playing a game of tennis, even a round of golf—as long as you walk the course and don't take a cart. Making a date and playing a game with a friend is a good way to increase the chances that you'll actually get out there and do it.

WHEN YOU FEEL BETTER, YOU'LL FEEL MORE LIKE MOVING

The good news is that people on the Alternate-Day Diet almost universally report feeling more energetic, as did the participants in our Asthma Study, and when you have more energy, you're also inclined to become more active.

George, for example, had suffered from severe asthma since the age of five. It was so severe that it had prevented him from joining the military. When he signed up for the study, his wheezing made him sound like a harmonica. His triglycerides were at 1064 milligrams per deciliter (normal is less than 150 mg/dL) and his blood looked as if there were globules of chicken fat floating on the surface. During the eight weeks of our study, not only did George lose 30 pounds but after just two weeks his triglycerides went down to 292 and the "chicken fat" disappeared. His asthma symptoms as well as his mood and energy levels also showed marked improvement. In fact, George felt so much better that he began to lift weights. His strength quickly increased and he reported feeling much more energetic on both the up and down days than he had before starting the diet.

Edna is another success story. When she first came to see me, she weighed 290 pounds and suffered from a constellation of more or less serious conditions including adult-onset asthma, Type 2 diabetes, toenail fungus, and impaired balance as the result of a bout with bacterial meningitis that had destroyed the hearing in her left ear. At the start of our study Edna was exhausted after walking 50 feet and found it almost impossible to climb a flight of stairs.

After just two weeks on the Alternate-Day Diet, she was experiencing a tremendous increase in energy. After four weeks, her asthma symptoms improved to the point where she was able to decrease the amount of medication she was taking. At the end of eight weeks she had lost 30 pounds, and her balance had improved so that she was able to walk easily and could even climb four flights of stairs. Her blood sugar levels returned to normal within ten weeks, her cholesterol and triglyceride levels declined dramatically, and and so did her markers for inflammation and

Get More Joy Out of Exercise

The most important characteristic of any exercise is how often you do it, and that depends on how much you enjoy it. Many people simply hate the idea of exercise in any form. To make it tolerable or even enjoyable, try the following.

For Cardio Training:

- If you start a walking program, don't pressure yourself to walk fast. Just show up, and over time you will automatically increase your speed and duration.

- Go to a park or a shopping mall where other people are walking. That way you won't feel alone.
- Find a workout partner with whom you meet at least one or two days a week. You are much more likely to show up if somebody else is expecting you.
- Use a Walkman or an iPod. Take the time to record the music you like or listen to an audiobook. Studies show that people do more exercise when listening to music with a personal listening device.
- On weekends, schedule a two-hour walk with a friend or a partner. Carry a backpack with some fixings to make it a picnic.
- Get a treadmill. Sturdy models are now available for less than $1,000.
- Watch TV while walking or running on the treadmill.

For Weight Training:

- Hire a trainer. A skilled trainer can get you started and keep you safe if you are new to strength training. Trainers can also provide essential encouragement and make sure that your form is correct.
- Go to a gym where there are other people. You are much more likely to actually work out if you're committed to a gym than if you stay at home.
- If you don't use a trainer, get a workout partner. Social interaction is perhaps the most important contributor to regularity of exercise. Use the Internet to find like-minded people.

oxidative damage. As a result of these marked improvements, Edna was literally transformed from a fatigued older woman to an energetic, joyful person who now loves walking several hours every day.

THE EFFECT IS SYNERGISTIC

When you're engaged in physical activity, you're also less likely to be thinking about being hungry. Have you ever noticed that when you're sitting on a plane for a long period of time, you tend to eat whatever food is offered—if it's offered—no matter how terrible it tastes? That's probably because you're bored and there isn't very much else for you to do. You've no doubt heard that when you're trying to diet and are tempted to eat you should engage in some kind of activity to take your mind off your stomach. The truth is, it works. When your mind and body are otherwise engaged, you're less likely to be eating or thinking about food. In fact, it's almost impossible to think about two things at once.

The bottom line is this: Any kind of physical activity has intrinsic health benefits, but it also has the ancillary benefit of giving you something to concentrate on other than your hunger—or your perception of hunger.

WHAT'S YOUR EXCUSE FOR NOT EXERCISING?

The biggest problem most people have with following any kind of exercise program is simply getting themselves to do it. It seems that we can be incredibly creative when it comes to thinking of reasons not to exercise.

The number one reason most people give for not exercising

is lack of time. I know that we're all very busy these days, but we seem to find time to do the things we *want* to do. Surely there are 30 minutes in your day when you could be getting some exercise if you weren't watching television or solving the crossword puzzle, or doing one of the other things that have so far kept you from exercising.

Other commonly perceived barriers to increasing physical activity are health concerns, weather, cost, and availability of facilities. All of these are really just other ways of saying that people simply don't believe they'll be able to organize and execute an exercise plan.

To overcome all these reasons *not to* exercise, it's of paramount importance that you understand and accept the reasons why you *should*. Regular exercise will:

- Increase lean muscle mass and reduce body fat.
- Help maintain healthy bones, muscles, and joints.
- Increase the number of calories you burn at rest (your RMR).
- Reduce your risk for coronary heart disease, high blood pressure, diabetes, and some cancers.
- Improve your mood and feelings of well-being.
- Increase mental alertness.

GATHER YOUR TOOLS— IT'S TIME TO GET STARTED

To recap:

- Determine your current calorie intake.
- Get yourself a journal and start to use it.

- Learn to read food labels.
- Make sure you have the proper measuring implements.
- Remember to drink (and eat) plenty of liquids.
- Exercise more.

Now turn the page and learn some of the basic nutritional principles that will enhance the effects of the Alternate-Day Diet.

7.

Nutrition: It's About Quantity and Quality

I've been saying all along that what you weigh is more important than what you eat for your overall health. I've also said that on the up day of the Alternate-Day Diet you will be eating freely, and I'm not going back on my word. After all, when I started the diet I didn't change the way I'd been eating on my up days. In terms of calories and weight loss, it's still *how much* you eat that counts. In terms of optimum health, however, the story may be a bit different. We now know that the foods we eat can significantly affect our risk for certain diseases, including heart disease, cancer, and Type 2 diabetes, and even though the evidence indicates that the Alternate-Day Diet will protect against these same diseases, I would be extremely remiss if I didn't provide you with some basic guidelines for good nutrition.

LIFE IS NOT A CLINICAL STUDY

I'm sure you've noticed that in our own Asthma Study, participants were allowed to eat whatever they wanted every other day and still saw the health benefits of alternate-day calorie restriction. We didn't specifically ask the participants in the study to report what they ate on their up days, but given that they were all overweight, it would be logical to assume that when left to their own devices, they weren't following a particularly healthy or calorie-reduced diet.

These studies, however, were just that—studies. They were time-limited, and as far as the animals were concerned, they could eat only what they were fed, which would have been a nutritious, species-specific diet.

The real point, however, is that, for you, the Alternate-Day Diet will be a way of life, something I hope you'll be doing from the day you start it. And it is not realistic to expect that all the people who start the Alternate-Day pattern will adhere to it perfectly for the rest of their lives. You won't be having calorie-controlled shakes on the down days every day. You probably won't be sticking to no more than 20 to 25 percent of your normal calorie intake on every down day forever. And you may be overeating on at least some of your up days. It would be great if you didn't, but it's simply not possible for anyone to be perfect. Therefore, it would be best to hedge your bets, so to speak, by eating as well as possible on as many days as possible.

By "eating well" I don't mean going to a fine-dining restaurant; I mean eating those foods that have been shown to promote good health and avoiding foods that are known to increase the risk of disease. For example, high-glycemic carbohydrates (white flour, rice, potatoes), saturated fat (beef, dairy), and foods prepared with trans fats (french fries, doughnuts) are clearly shown to be contributors to heart disease.

According to Walter Willett, by following an optimal diet

combined with a healthy lifestyle (which includes maintaining a healthy weight, exercising, and not smoking) we could eliminate 80 percent of heart attacks, 70 percent of strokes, more than 90 percent of Type 2 diabetes, and more than 70 percent of colon cancer. In other words, the world's foremost nutritional authority is telling us a major cause of all these conditions is *what* we eat. It would be foolish of anyone to ignore those statistics.

NOTHING IS FORBIDDEN

Without minimizing the many benefits of following a healthy diet, my colleagues and I believe, on the basis of the Asthma Study diet, that if your calorie intake is low enough on the down days, you can eat anything you want to on the up days and still have remarkable health benefits. So I am not going to give you a list of forbidden foods. That would be the ultimate bait-and-switch, and it would also be highly unrealistic. But while no foods are forbidden on the up days of this diet, there are foods you should be eating more often, because they will help to promote good health, and others that should be eaten less often and with the understanding that they could compromise your health over time.

WHAT TO EAT FOR OPTIMAL NUTRITION

I'm sure you've heard it before: Eat a diet based on whole grains, fruits and leafy green vegetables, plant-based fats, and lean protein. Avoid sugary, starchy, refined carbohydrates, red meat, full-fat dairy, and trans fats. But you may have had trouble trans-lating that advice into practical terms. The following information is designed to help you do that.

The True Skinny on Fat

Does eating fat make you fat and put you at greater risk for heart disease? Depending on how much as well as what kind of fat you eat, both parts of that statement may be true. But fat is also essential for building cell membranes and the protective sheaths surrounding your nerves. It is necessary for making certain hormones, controlling blood clotting, and regulating muscle contraction—including the contractions of your heart. We all need some fat in our diet, but not all fats are the same, and not all fats are equally healthy.

What Are Fats Made of, and Why Do I Care?

All types of fat are made of a chain of carbon atoms bonded to hydrogen atoms. When a fat is saturated, it means that the carbon atoms hold as many hydrogen atoms as they can. Each carbon atom is connected to its neighbors on either side by a single bond. Examined under a microscope, saturated fats look like straight chains. You probably don't examine your food under a microscope, but one way you can recognize a saturated fat is by the fact that it congeals and is solid at room temperature—like butter or bacon fat or the fat encircling and marbling a steak.

It's saturated fat that's primarily responsible for clogging up our arteries and raising our levels of LDL (bad) cholesterol. But not even all saturated fats are the same. You may be surprised to know that the saturated fat in butter and whole-fat dairy products has more of a worse effect on cholesterol than beef fat, and the fats in chocolate and cocoa butter have less. Regardless, saturated fats raise LDL (bad cholesterol) and have little effect on HDL (good cholesterol).

When a fat is monounsaturated, at one point along the chain two carbon atoms are connected by a double bond. This change reduces by two the number of hydrogen atoms the chain can hold and changes the shape from straight to bent. Monounsaturated fats are liquid at room temperature. In other words, they're oils. Olive, peanut, and canola oils are all high in monounsaturated fat, and avocados as well as most nuts are also good sources.

When a fat has two or more double bonds, it is polyunsaturated and can hold even fewer hydrogen atoms. These fats look like sticks with two bends. They are divided into two categories: omega-3 and omega-6, and the main difference between them and monounsaturated fats is that our body can't make them. We must get our polyunsaturated fats from dietary sources or supplements. The best dietary sources of these essential fats are fatty fish like tuna and salmon, as well as plant sources like corn and soybean oil, soy and soy products, and seeds.

Both monounsaturated and polyunsaturated fats lower LDL and raise HDL.

The healthiest balance between polyunsaturated and monounsaturated fat has not been established, but monounsaturated fat appears to confer greater protection against fatal heart rhythm disturbances, the commonest cause of death in heart attacks.

The last type of fat, trans fat (sometimes called partially hydrogenated vegetable oil), should be avoided as much as possible. A small amount of trans fat is present in animal fat, but most of what we consume is artificial.

About a hundred years ago, chemists discovered that they could solidify vegetable oil by heating it in the presence of hydrogen gas. Their discovery is what gave us products like margarine and Crisco. It also allowed food manufacturers to create products with a longer shelf life. At one time, it was thought that trans fats were healthier than the saturated fat found in butter, but studies since the 1970s have shown that trans fats have an even greater effect on raising levels of LDL (bad cholesterol) and creating artery-clogging plaque than saturated fat. Plus, they *lower* levels of HDL (good cholesterol), which saturated fat doesn't do. Recently, the food industry has gotten the message, and the trans fat picture is steadily improving. Many margarines have been reformulated to contain zero or less than 0.5g per serving of trans fat, but you should always check the label. According to the Institute of Medicine, doughnuts and french fries are probably the commonest sources of trans fats in our diet, but many baked goods also have large quantities.

Healthy Fats Reduce Your Risk for Dying of a Heart Attack

The results of the Lyon Diet Heart Study, a randomized, controlled trial that considered the effectiveness of a Mediterranean-type diet, indicate the dramatic effect of changing from a predominantly saturated animal-fat diet to a diet low in saturated fat and high in monounsaturated and polyunsaturated fats. In the study, all participants had survived a first heart attack. The experimental group—302 men and women—were put on a healthy-fat Mediterranean-type diet and compared with a control group of 303 people with similar coronary risk factors who received no specific dietary advice but were asked by their physician to eat prudently. The study was actually discontinued earlier than planned, because the results showed that those following the healthy-fat diet had a 70 percent lower risk of recurrent heart disease than the control group following the traditional diet.

Monounsaturated and polyunsaturated fats stabilize the electrical conduction system in the heart, thereby preventing the abnormal heart rhythms that are a leading cause of cardiac deaths. But you don't have to have a heart attack before you change from saturated to monounsaturated and polyunsaturated fat!

DECODING CARBOHYDRATES

Basically, carbohydrates are the nutrients that most significantly affect your blood sugar levels. All the carbohydrates you eat are digested and broken down to sugar, but some turn to sugar more quickly than others. The best way to differentiate one type of carbohydrate from another is by how rapidly they raise your blood sugar. The glycemic index was created by nutrition researcher David Jenkins and his colleagues at the University of Toronto to measure the speed and degree to which various carbohydrates raise blood sugar levels. Foods that are high on the glycemic index raise the blood sugar level more than those that are low on the index. As a general rule, foods containing large quantities of sugar, starches (including white rice, potatoes, crackers, and most white breads), and baked goods made with refined flour have a high GI rating.

You may have heard carbohydrates referred to as simple or complex. Generally speaking, complex carbohydrates are those with a low glycemic index number, such as whole grains and vegetables. These contain important nutrients called phytochemicals that protect against free-radical damage and oxidative stress. They are also the primary source of dietary fiber, which performs a variety of important functions.

Basically, fiber—what your parents probably called roughage—is required for healthy bowel function. Fiber absorbs water like a sponge and creates bulk, which allows the gut to propel the food onward. It protects against constipation, diverticulosis, and diverticulitis.

There are two kinds of fiber, soluble and insoluble. Soluble fiber dissolves, of course, and it forms a gelatinous mass. It traps bile acids and lowers cholesterol. Good sources of soluble fiber include apples, citrus fruits, peas, and oats. Insoluble fiber, from the cell walls of plants, consists of long chains of glucose molecules that our GI tract can't break down or dissolve. The chief sources of insoluble fiber are fruits, vegetables, and whole grains.

At one time, insoluble fiber was thought to prevent cancer of the colon, but recent large studies have failed to support this theory. It is, however, valuable in reducing the absorption of sugar and starch, thereby lessening glucose-insulin spikes in the

Get More Whole Grains in Your Diet

What makes a whole grain "whole" is that none of its components have been removed in processing. The components of the grain are either intact, as with brown rice or whole oats, or, if it has been processed by grinding, all of the components are retained. The two elements that are removed in refined white wheat flour, for example, are the bran (fiber) and the wheat germ, both of which are important for preventing a variety of diseases. Whole grains not only help to reduce body weight but also reduce the incidence of stroke, Type 2 diabetes, heart disease, inflammatory disease, diverticulitis, and constipation. Whole grains *may* also help reduce the incidence of colorectal cancer, high blood pressure, and periodontitis (gum disease).

The recommended daily consumption is six servings per day, although one (half-cup) serving per day reduces disease risk; generally speaking, the more the better. To get more whole grains in your diet try:

- Breakfast grains: whole oats (groats), steel-cut oats, rolled long-cooking oats, oatmeal, Wheaties, Wheat Chex, Grape-Nuts, All-Bran, shredded wheat, and Kashi multigrain cereals
- Brown rice
- Pearl barley (have it as a side dish with a light vinaigrette, add it to soups or salads, or try it in chili or with beans instead of rice)
- Whole-grain crackers: Triscuits, Wheat Thin Multi Grains, Kashi TLC, chips
- Whole-grain breads: The *first* ingredient listed must say *whole* for a bread to be a whole-grain bread, but multigrain breads are better than plain white bread
- Whole-wheat pasta

bloodstream, which in turn helps to reduce heart disease and Type 2 diabetes.

WHAT YOU SHOULD KNOW ABOUT GLYCEMIC LOAD

To take the glycemic index to the next level, so to speak, and to better reflect the effect of various carbohydrates on blood sugar, Walter Willett and his colleagues at the Department of Nutrition, Harvard School of Public Health, developed another scale called the glycemic load, which takes into account not only the glycemic index rating of various foods but also the *amount* of carbohydrates in the food. Carrots, for example, are high on the glycemic index, but carrots also have a high water content, which means that, gram for gram, they deliver only a small amount of carbohydrates, do not create a rapid rise in blood sugar, and therefore have a low glycemic load.

The overall goal is to understand which foods, and what quantities of those foods, to select or avoid on the basis of their glycemic

Can Food Be Addictive?

"Are there certain things in food that act on the brain and set up a classic addictive process, like tolerance, withdrawal and craving?" asks psychologist Kelly Brownell of Yale University. The evidence is mounting that food addiction is real.

Addiction to drugs is manifested by changes in the brain that can be seen in MRIs, and abstinence and recovery from drug addiction produce a return to normal patterns. We believe that avoidance of high-sugar, high-fat foods by eating a diet high in vegetables can produce recovery of these brain mechanisms.

Using MRI brain imaging, psychiatrist Nora D. Volkow and her colleagues at Brookhaven National Laboratory have shown that, like amphetamine addicts, obese people have fewer receptors for dopamine, and the higher the body mass index, the fewer the dopamine receptors. The dopamine system in the brain is what is stimulated when we experience any pleasurable feeling—such as we get from eating or sex. The dopamine systems of drug addicts are overstimulated, and the withdrawal and craving they experience result from these receptors crying out for more of the drug. The craving overpowers the will of the addict, who is unable to stop using the drug.

It appears that some people may have a greater rise in dopamine levels in response to high-sugar, high-fat foods and may become "addicted" to these foods. The rapid return of "hunger" after eating high-glycemic foods may, therefore, result not simply from a drop in blood sugar from the overrelease of insulin but may indicate a deficiency of the "food drug" that causes these people to think about food in the same way addicts think about drugs.

People in developing countries whose diets are low in fat and sugar do not seem to experience these same food cravings. This could be because their dopamine receptors haven't been damaged by high-sugar, high-fat foods, and Dr. Laub's and my clinical experience suggests that following a diet that avoids these foods on the up days will, over time, reduce our thoughts about and cravings for food.

index and glycemic load. You can find a comprehensive list of both the GI and GL of various foods at mendosa.com/gilists.htm.

Mix Up Your Fruits and Vegetables

Plant foods contain a variety of phytonutrients ("phyto" meaning plant-based). Accumulating research indicates that many chronic diseases may be partially caused by a relative deficiency of these plant substances. In fact, it is now well established that eating a diet high in fruits and vegetables results in lower rates of heart disease, stroke, high blood pressure, cataracts and macular degeneration, cancer (see the box on the following page), Type 2 diabetes, Alzheimer's disease, and decline in thinking skills. For this reason, the Food and Drug Administration now recommends that we eat nine half-cup servings of a wide variety of fruits and vegetables every day.

Among those that have been studied most extensively and whose health benefits are well documented are broccoli, tomatoes (preferably cooked), spinach, onions and garlic, and carrots. I recommend that you make these your "first choice" vegetables and eat them several times a week as part of the Alternate-Day Diet.

The broader categories of fruits and vegetables to include in your diet are as follows:

- *Cruciferous:* broccoli, cauliflower, Brussels sprouts, cabbage, turnips, and rutabaga. They provide isothiocyanates, folate, calcium, iron, and vitamin K, which protects against cancer.
- *Melon/squash family:* cucumbers, zucchini, pumpkin, winter squash, and cantaloupe. Orange members of this group are rich in carotenes.

- *Solanum family* (actually a genus): tomatoes (rich in lycopene), peppers, and eggplant.
- *Umbels:* carrots (beta-carotene), parsnips, and parsley.
- *Lily family:* Onions, garlic, leeks, shallots, and asparagus, which contain sulfur compounds (allicin, diallyl sulfate) that may fight cancer.
- *Legume family:* beans, peas, and soybeans, all of which contain folate, fiber, and protease inhibitors, which protect against heart disease and cancer.
- *Citrus family:* lemons, limes, oranges, and grapefruit. These contain vitamin C and limonene, which have anti-cancer properties.
- *All dark-colored berries (blue, red, black),* which are rich in antioxidants and pigmented polyphenols.

Do Fruits and Vegetables Really Protect Against Cancer?

It is clear that lifestyle choices—including smoking, drinking excess alcohol, inactivity, and obesity—are associated with a higher chance of developing cancer, and the expert consensus is that a diet rich in fruits and vegetables may reduce the risk of esophageal, stomach, lung, mouth, throat, ovarian, kidney, bladder, and colorectal cancer. That said, however, the best available data does *not* show that a diet high in vegetables and fruit reduces the *overall incidence* of cancer. On the other hand, the accumulated science in calorie restriction shows that it *does prevent* cancer in animals and humans. Studies in every-other-day feeding show that cancer rates are lowered.

PICKING THE RIGHT PROTEINS

Protein is made up of approximately twenty basic components called amino acids that are the building blocks of our cells, and we need all of them to stay alive. Some forms of protein, called complete proteins, contain all of these amino acids. Other foods provide only some and need to be eaten in combination in order to ensure that we are getting all the amino acids we need. Complete proteins are derived from animal sources including meat, poultry, fish, eggs, dairy products, and soy. As a rule, vegetable sources provide incomplete proteins.

According to the latest dietary guidelines, we need to eat about 7 grams of protein for every 20 pounds of body weight, but

What's So Great About Soy?

Soy has the reputation of being beneficial for lowering cholesterol, but this idea is based on a study in which lower cholesterol levels were found in people who ate 50 grams of soy per day instead of animal protein sources (which contain saturated fat). In order to get enough to match the study, you would have to eat a pound of tofu every day (not a good idea), and later studies have not shown any effect of soy on cholesterol. Menopause-related hot flashes may be helped by soy, but the evidence is weak, as is evidence supporting the effect of soy in decreasing incidence of breast cancer and heart disease.

In the words of Harvard's Walter Willett, soy "may have a dark side." In fact, estrogen-sensitive breast cancer may be adversely affected by soy, which has its own estrogenic properties and can interfere with tamoxifen, an important breast cancer treatment drug. Seventh-day Adventist women, who are vegetarian and eat soy, show a rising rate of breast cancer the longer they are vegetarian. The claim that breast cancer occurs less in Japanese women because they eat soy is clearly wrong. Breast cancer is rare throughout Asia, but most Asian populations do not eat soy.

In addition, there is evidence that decline in cognitive function, memory loss, and age-related brain atrophy may be worse in older men who eat more than two servings of tofu per week. Finally, there is also uncertainty about the effect of soy on prostate cancer.

These persistent negative indications lead me to recommend that you eat soy products a few times per week at most.

The Atkins Diet Fallacy

As far back as 1972, Robert Atkins was advocating eating a high-protein, low-carbohydrate diet for weight loss. It took nearly thirty years before medical scientists began to study his claims that people lose weight faster and with less hunger on this diet. Although he was not the first to advocate this scheme, his name has now become synonymous with the diet that allows you to eat unlimited amounts of steaks, burgers, eggs, and dairy products. But the lack of sufficient fruits and vegetables, whole grains, and cereal fiber, along with the unlimited consumption of saturated fat, fly in the face of the new science of nutrition.

More recently, the South Beach Diet has advocated healthier sources of protein in the form of fish and fowl, both of which provide healthier fats than red meat.

There is evidence from a variety of sources that both Atkins and South Beach work for short-term weight loss. One year after starting a diet, however, there appears to be no significant difference in success rate than that seen on any other common diet plan. If the overall test of whether a diet "works" is the degree to which people voluntarily adopt the plan, lose weight, and maintain the weight loss in a free-living environment, it is evident that no diet has yet been successful.

The Mayo Clinic studied the citizens of Multnomah County, Oregon, and found that they were more aware of the Atkins Diet than other diets and would use it as a first choice for weight loss. The problem was that the population as a whole was gaining weight, just as the rest of the country was. This may be because people who are in a chronic state of attempting to stick with high-protein foods become hungry for carbohydrates. So they order the largest steak on the menu and then have some dessert anyway. If they followed the Atkins Diet for a discrete period to lose a specific amount of weight and then switched to a nutritionally healthy diet, it might be a good way to lose weight. But they are no more able to sustain the high-protein pattern over time than they are to comply with any diet that requires the daily restriction of amount or type of food.

Protein may, indeed, help to increase satiety or satiation (the period of time until hunger returns), and there may also be value in the ketosis created by eating a primarily noncarbohydrate diet. (The Alternate-Day Diet also produces ketosis—elevated hydroxy butyrate—which appears to increase the brain's resistance to stress and may also contribute to suppression of hunger.)

That said, however, no diet that requires the consumption or restriction of any particular macronutrient or component will produce long-term weight loss, because all of the factors that determine appetite are too powerful and overwhelm our conscious effort to control our eating.

for the most part, no one should really have to think about getting enough protein—it's almost impossible not to. The only issue would be for strict vegetarians to eat enough variety to be certain that they are getting all the various amino acids they require.

It's What You Get Along with Your Protein That Counts

Except for simple sugars, almost no food comprises just one nutrient. So while pretty much all kinds of protein are equally healthy, what comes along with them is not. Beef, for example, is a great source of complete protein, but it comes bound up with a lot of unhealthy, saturated animal fat. Poultry and fish are also complete proteins, and the fat they contain is mainly unsaturated, which makes them much healthier sources than red meat. Full-fat dairy products, because they come from animals (cows, sheep, and goats), are also high in saturated fat.

In terms of fat content, plant proteins—including nuts, seeds, legumes, vegetables, and grains—are the healthiest choices of all, as long as you eat enough variety to ensure that no essential amino acids are missing from your diet.

What Does a Healthy Meal Look Like?

Well, it could look like a lot of different things. How about a bowl of whole-wheat pasta with marinara sauce, a piece of whole-wheat bread dipped in olive oil, and a green salad with vinaigrette dressing? Here are a few other healthy up-day choices you may not have considered:

Turkey burger on a whole-wheat bun (with ketchup, mayonnaise made with olive or soybean oil, and a slice of onion)
An ear of corn
Salad made with romaine lettuce, reduced-fat blue cheese, and olive-oil-and-vinegar dressing

Chicken breast dipped in egg white and whole-wheat bread crumbs sautéed in olive oil
Baked sweet potato
Grilled asparagus with a squirt of lemon juice

Poached salmon
Cucumber salad
Brown rice

Tuna packed in olive oil
Mixed with cooked white (cannellini) beans and seasoned with chopped fresh basil and/or Italian parsley

Eggs Are Really Okay

Despite the American Egg Board's ongoing promotion of the "incredible edible egg," eggs have been getting a bad rap for years. But according to nutritionist Walter Willett, "Eggs aren't just packets of cholesterol. They are very low in saturated fat and contain many other nutrients that are good for you. . . . So their effect on heart disease risk can't be predicted by considering only their cholesterol content. . . . No research has ever shown that people who eat more eggs have more heart attacks than people who eat few eggs. . . . The most comprehensive study to date looked at the egg-eating habits of almost 120,000 men and women. Healthy men and women who ate up to an egg a day were no more likely to have developed heart disease or to have had a stroke over many years of follow-up than those who ate less than one egg a week."

Egg white vegetable omelet cooked in vegetable oil
Whole-wheat toast

Notice that I haven't given any quantities for the above choices. Your up days are not about restricting calories (although stuffing yourself is not a good idea either) but about choosing to get the calories you do eat from healthier sources.

In Chapter 9, I'll be giving you lists of various foods with portion sizes and calorie counts to keep you on track during your down days. For a selection of healthy, nutritious down-day menus and recipes, go to Chapter 11.

Should You Take Dietary Supplements?
If So, Which Ones, and Why?

It has been estimated that the DNA in each of our cells sustains 10,000 injuries per day from free radicals. The resulting damage can in rare cases result in cancer or other life-threatening illnesses. Our main defense against this kind of damage lies with the thousands of antioxidants we get from food and dietary supplements that neutralize free radicals.

Among the most common known antioxidants are vitamins C and E, beta-carotene and other carotenoids, selenium, and manganese. Other antioxidants now being studied with growing interest are glutathione, coenzyme Q10, alpha-lipoic acid, flavonoids, polyphenols, and phytoestrogens. Every type of antioxidant plays a slightly different role in the elaborate protective mechanism, and for that reason it is important to consume all the different types that are found in a healthy diet.

Many studies have shown that it's both safer and more effective to get your vitamins and antioxidants from food sources than from pills. In fact, according to the most recent analysis of prospective randomized trials of antioxidant supplements, beta-carotene, vitamin A, and vitamin E were associated with higher mortality rates, and vitamin C and selenium showed no benefit. Overall, the authors of the analysis estimated a 5 percent increase in mortality—caused mainly by cancer and heart disease—among people taking antioxidant supplements.

Some studies, however, do support the value of some antioxidant supplements. For example, in the Nurses' Health Study and the Health Professionals Follow-Up Study, vitamin E *tended* to reduce the incidence of heart disease, although the difference was not statistically significant. And there is also some weak evidence supporting cancer reduction in men taking antioxidant supplements.

The antioxidant effect of two carotenoids—lutein and zeaxanthin—probably help slow the progression of macular degeneration, the commonest cause of blindness in older people. These are available in supplements whose label indicates that they are for "eye health."

Further trials will be necessary to determine whether or not taking supplements of single antioxidants is of value for reducing disease.

It appears to be particularly dangerous to take high doses of vitamins. Men taking more than seven multivitamin pills per week showed a severalfold increase in advanced and fatal prostate cancer, although the overall *incidence* of prostate cancer did not change, meaning that some cases of localized prostate cancer were transformed into advanced and fatal cancer. And the overall incidence of prostate cancer was also increased in men who took selenium, folic acid, or vitamin E along with their multivitamins.

A number of other studies have also shown risks for taking vitamins in doses above the recommended daily allowance (RDA).

That said, however, there are some vitamins we don't get enough of even from the most nutritious diet. Among these are three of the B vitamins—B_9 (folic acid), B_6, and B_{12} all of which may reduce the risk for heart disease and cancer. They help to recycle homocysteine, a byproduct of eating protein, by turning it into amino acids instead of allowing it to build up and clog the arteries. High levels of homocysteine have been shown to increase the risk of heart disease. All three of these B vitamins are available in multivitamin capsules.

Unlike the B vitamins, however, vitamin D—which helps the

body to absorb calcium, protects the skin against sun damage, and has been shown to reduce the incidence of various cancers—is not found in high enough doses in multivitamins. It is present in the diet and is produced in the skin in response to sun, but to reap its anticancer benefits most people require at least 1,000 IU (international units) a day, which requires taking a separate pill. People over the age of seventy should take more than younger people. A large meta-analysis recently showed that optimal treatment with vitamin D would prevent 250,000 cases of colorectal cancer and 350,000 cases of breast cancer worldwide. The researchers' recommendation was to take 2,000 IU per day and spend 15 to 20 minutes in the sun exposing 40 percent of your skin. A blood test to measure 25-hydroxy vitamin D is the best way to know if you are getting the right dose. Taking vitamin D supplements is one of the most important steps you can take to reduce your likelihood of cancer.

Calcium may also require supplementation if you are receiving less than 500 mg per day through dietary sources. Contrary to what many people believe, dairy products—because they are high in calories and saturated fat—are not the best sources of dietary calcium. Some good nondairy food sources of calcium include dark-green leafy vegetables, fish (including salmon, sardines, and ocean perch), and tofu.

Determining whether or not to take supplements and which ones to choose can be a confusing and daunting prospect. Although some could be beneficial, others might well be unnecessary or even detrimental to your health. The supplement industry is largely unregulated, and manufacturers are allowed to suggest all kinds of health benefits whether or not they've been proved. In fact, they are not even required to guarantee that the ingredients stated on the label accurately reflect what you're getting in the bottle. And yet approximately half of all adult Americans are taking one or more supplements to benefit their health.

The following are supplements that have established scientific evidence to recommend them; just be sure that if you do decide to take one or more of them, you choose a brand from a reputable manufacturer. When it comes to your health, it's not a good idea to pinch pennies.

Omega-3 Fatty Acids: These essential polyunsaturated fatty acids, which your body cannot manufacture, play important roles in cellular function, especially in the brain, and are necessary for maintaining a normal heart rhythm. To be sure you are getting a sufficient supply you would need to eat about 12 ounces of fatty fish per week. A simpler and perhaps safer source, given the mercury content of some fish, is fish oil capsules, which are made with oil from fatty fish that's been purified to remove mercury and other toxins. Fish oil capsules are available at drugstores, grocery stores, and discount and large-box stores. The dose that appears to confer protection from cardiovascular disease, mainly by preventing fatal heart rhythms, is three 1-gram capsules per day, each containing 180 mg of eicosapentaenoic acid and 120 mg of docosahexaenoic acid. Higher doses probably don't improve heart health.

For rheumatoid arthritis, you'd need to take ten capsules a day to get the anti-inflammatory effect.

Alpha-Lipoic Acid: Alpha-lipoic acid affects age-related mitochondrial function and may, therefore, treat a variety of age-related health problems, including heart disease, diabetes, Alzheimer's, diminished muscle strength, and decline in brain function. In combination with acetyl-L-carnitine (see below), it has been shown to reverse cognitive decline in old rats, and human studies are now under way. Because your body does not manufacture it, you need to take supplements in order to get its potentially powerful antioxidant benefits. The usual recommended daily dose is 800 mg taken as 400 mg twice a day.

Acetyl-L-carnitine (ALCAR): This mitochondrial "food" when taken in combination with alpha-lipoic acid restores age-related damage to mitochondria, which translates as improvement in cognitive function. A number of randomized controlled trials have shown significant improvement in cognitive impairment and mild Alzheimer's disease, as well as in diabetic neuropathy.

Coenzyme Q10: This supplement is recommended for people with high blood pressure, those taking statin drugs, those with risk factors for heart disease, and older people in general. Published reports indicate that a dose of up to 1,200 mg per day (taken as 400 mg three times a day) has beneficial effects on lowering blood pressure and reducing migraine headaches, and may protect against heart attack and neurodegenerative brain disorders such as Parkinson's.

THE BOTTOM LINE

Following the Alternate-Day Diet will help you to lose weight and live longer. Making sure the majority of the foods you eat on your up day are nutritious and healthful will enhance its protective effects, and taking a few supplements that have been scientifically proved to reduce or reverse the effects of age-related illnesses will keep you even healthier longer.

Calorie restriction is the most powerful potential mechanism to improve human health and the Alternate-Day Diet makes the application of this theory possible for most people.

8.

Step 1:
The Induction Phase

This is the most restrictive phase of the diet, but it lasts only two weeks. Two weeks isn't very long—especially when the restriction is limited to every other day, which means a total of only seven days!

During this time you will be restricting your down-day calorie intake to no more than 20 percent of what you would normally eat. To simplify matters for you, I've rounded this off to 500 calories, which is about 20 percent of the total calories eaten daily by the average overweight woman. I arrived at that number based on a couple of criteria. First, if you consume 20 percent of your normal calories on alternate days, you will be reducing your total calorie consumption by 40 percent a day (a total reduction of 80 percent—on the down day—spread over a two-day period), which means that, on average, you'll be eating 60 percent of what you would eat normally, which is the figure that has been shown by various studies to be maximally effective in prolonging the lifespan of a number of species. And second, I thought—and later proved through the Asthma Study as well as my own experience and that of others who have tried it—that eating 20 percent of what they normally would every other day is tolerable for most people.

Use a Meal-Replacement Shake to Control Down-Day Calories

For the first two weeks, you will be getting your 500 down-day calories specifically from meal-replacement shakes such as Slim Fast, Ensure, Atkins, and Zone, to name the most popular and widely available. In fact, if you don't use the shakes in place of regular food on your first two weeks of down days, you will probably not be successful. This statement is based not only on my own experience and that of my patients but also on the many studies of meal-replacement shakes that confirm their usefulness in helping people adhere to their intended intake.

There are several reasons for this.

- Accuracy: The meal-replacement shake makes it easy to determine how many calories you are actually consuming.

  Eating regular food on a down day is likely to allow denial and rationalization to creep in. Studies have shown most people are not capable of accurately judging how much they eat because the powerful survival instinct to eat overwhelms our conscious intentions. One of the main reasons people fail at diets is the rationalization that unconsciously allows us to lie to ourselves about how much we are consuming.
- You won't have to think about what you're going to eat next, which means that you won't be thinking about food

all the time. Soon you will notice that you have far fewer thoughts about food on your down days.

- Because these drinks, while certainly palatable, are not generally "taste treats," you won't be tempted to have more than you should just because it tastes good, so you'll be much more likely to eat (or drink) only when you're actually hungry, which will also give you a better sense of what hunger actually feels like.
- Shakes are portable and easy to carry with you throughout the day so that you can have a sip when you feel overwhelmed by hunger.

Canned shakes vary in protein, fat, and carbohydrate content. Those that are lowest in carbohydrates and sugar are preferable because a higher sugar content will stimulate insulin, which turns off SIRT1. But the amount of sugar in the shake is less important than the total calories you consume, so find the one that is most palatable for you.

Making the Most of Your Shake

Rather than consuming your entire shake all at once, you'll be drinking small amounts (1 to 5 ounces at a time) throughout the day and evening. This will minimize not only your feelings of hunger but also your body's reaction to the calories, and thus will help to intensify the SIRT1 gene-activating mechanism.

WHAT TO EXPECT ON THE DOWN DAYS

Your first down day will certainly be the hardest. At first you may think that it will be impossible for you to get through the day on just 20 percent of what you've been eating. Then, after you have 100 or 200 calories in the form of a shake for breakfast and again for lunch, you'll realize that although you may not be full, you are not starving, and you actually feel good. This will undoubtedly come as a delightful surprise.

The real temptation invariably comes between 11 a.m. and 2:30 p.m., when you feel you have to eat in order to perform optimally. But, as you'll discover after just a few days, you really don't *need* to eat.

By late afternoon you'll undoubtedly be assaulted by both hunger and fatigue. When this happens, you can restore yourself with a few minutes' rest and/or meditation, drinking water to rehydrate yourself, and another 100 calories from your shake.

Dinnertime can also be a challenge because sharing a meal is so much a part of the social ritual. You can, however, participate in the social interaction even if you're only drinking the shake.

The hours between dinner and bedtime may be the most challenging of all, because you won't be distracted by work or other daily activities. It's important to have a procedure to follow when the pressure to eat seems to be too great: Sit down, close your eyes, take four deep breaths, inhale/exhale slowly, visualize your thin body enjoying yourself, remind yourself why you are doing this, and recite the Alternate-Day mantras ("I'll eat tomorrow," "Don't blow it," "Get busy," "It's worth it."). Get outside yourself by engaging someone else (help your children with their homework, etc.), call a supportive friend or relative, or engage yourself in some simple, repetitive task.

Save 100 or 200 calories for bedtime to help you fall asleep, and go to bed early. Most of us are sleep-deprived anyway.

After just three or four days, you'll notice that you don't feel as hungry, your down days will become easier—in fact, you'll actually begin to look forward to how you feel, because you'll be experiencing an improvement in energy and mood. Alternate-Day dieters often describe this as feeling "wired," "euphoric," "like being in love," or "like the Energizer Bunny."

Additionally, the alternate-day eating pattern appears to create an unconscious habit that suppresses thoughts of hunger and food. The universal experience of those on the diet is that they are much less aware of hunger or thoughts about food, so, in effect, their perceived hunger is greatly reduced. In other words, just as practice builds muscle memory when you're learning to play a sport, our minds learn to not think about what we have made a decision not to think about.

DOWN-DAY STRATEGIES TO STAVE OFF HUNGER

I'm not saying that you won't ever be hungry on your down days. But your down days are only 24 hours long, and, it is hoped, for about 8 of those hours you'll be sleeping. There are, however, some simple strategies you can use to stay strong when you think you're going to blow it.

- When you *think* you must eat, wait a few minutes. More often than not, the craving will have passed. Hunger pangs occur in waves every 2 to 3 hours and typically last 15 to 20 minutes. Remind yourself that the hunger will go away if you can distract yourself for that short period of time.
- If you still think you're hungry, take a sip of your shake.

After you've had a couple of sips, your hunger will probably be alleviated.

- Drink calorie-free liquids as much as you want on the down day to avoid becoming dehydrated, which can make you feel weak and tired and make you think you're hungry. Many of us tend to think we're hungry when we're really just thirsty. And the water will also fill you up for a while. As a guideline, drink at least 2 liters of calorie-free liquid in addition to the shake. Coffee, diet colas, and the like are okay (in fact, caffeine may raise your blood sugar slightly and reduce feelings of hunger), but it is best not to take in too much caffeine: it may make you feel overstimulated because of the energizing effect of the diet.
- Get involved in an activity you enjoy that occupies your mind and your hands. It's hard to think about two things at once, and if your hands are busy, you won't be using them to eat.
- Call somebody. Mutual support helps you to stay with the program.
- Sit down, close your eyes, and tell yourself to relax. Take four deep breaths, exhaling slowly, and rest for 5 minutes.
- Visualize yourself thin, enjoying yourself, and recite the reasons you are following the diet: to enjoy better health, to live longer, to feel happy about the way you look.
- Use the following aphorisms to boost your resolve:

  - I will eat tomorrow, or I can always eat tomorrow.
  - Put off until tomorrow what you can't eat today.
  - It's the calories, stupid!
  - It's not the carbs, it's the calories, sweetie!
  - Rx Food: Take only as directed.

- Surgeon general's warning: Overeating may be injurious to your health.
- If not now, when?
- I'll be around for my family.
- It's worth it!

WHAT ABOUT THE UP DAYS?

This is the part you want to hear: On the up days eat anything you want. Particularly when you start the diet, it's important to feel that you can have anything you want to eat every other day so that you avoid the sense of deprivation that sets in with other diets. Remember, compliance is everything, and most people who tend to be overweight have tried numerous diets, have developed a sense of frustration and failure, and envision the future as an infinite horizon of hunger and deprivation. The up days on this diet are your insurance that no matter what you're feeling today, you can always eat tomorrow. And if you're sticking to 20 percent of normal calorie intake on your down days, you'd have to eat a whopping 180 percent on your up days just to come out even. As a practical matter, this just doesn't happen, at least in the first three months or so.

As time passes, however, people do begin to increase their up day intake, with a resultant slowing of weight loss. At that point it's a good idea to begin keeping a record of your up-day intake to become more mindful of what you are eating. You still need to be aware of the hungry crocodile within and remain conscious of when you're eating for pleasure rather than because you're hungry.

In our Asthma Study there was some evidence that the subjects were restraining themselves (but to a far less degree) on the

How Much Can You Expect to Lose?

You can estimate your projected weekly weight loss by assuming that all weight-loss results from a reduction in body fat—although, particularly in the first week or so, you will experience several pounds of water loss, and some of the weight loss that occurs over time may be due to muscle loss. As a rough estimate, however, a pound of fat supplies 3,500 calories, the amount by which you must reduce your intake to lose one pound. So if your estimated daily calorie requirement is 2,000, over 30 days you require 60,000 calories to maintain your weight. If you consume 20 percent, or 400 calories on 15 down days, and 2,000 calories on 15 up days, your calorie intake for the 30 days is 15 x 2,000 + (15 x 400) = 36,000 calories. Therefore, 60,000 − 36,000 (24,000) is your calorie deficit, and 24,000 ÷ 3,500 = 6.9 pounds of fat lost in 30 days.

up days as well as on the down days. This is a natural consequence of the desire to lose weight and there is no harm in restraining to some degree on the up day. It is critically important, however, that you not feel deprived; otherwise the Alternate-Day Diet would be nothing more than another daily dieting program. The goal is to eat whatever you want until you're satisfied, but not to overeat.

WHAT TO EXPECT ON THE UP DAYS

When you wake up after your first down day your initial thought will undoubtedly be something like "Wow! I did it!" You'll be amazed that you were able to limit yourself to only 500 calories, and you'll be proud of your achievement. You'll also realize that you aren't hungry—or at least not any hungrier than you would normally be.

Within just a few days you'll begin to realize that hunger is not the overwhelming force you imagined it to be. You'll start to feel proud of your ability to conquer the dragon of hunger. This is the central realization that makes it possible to continue the Alternate-Day Diet feeling hopeful and reborn.

Within a short time you'll begin to see that your attitude toward food, even on the up days, has changed. You'll eat to satisfaction, but you won't overeat as you might have done before you began the diet. You'll actually want to feel slightly empty rather than too full.

Interestingly, your food preferences will also start to change. You'll begin to think, "Oh boy, I can eat whatever I want! But what I want is not what I thought I'd want." The compulsion to eat something "bad" (say a dozen Krispy Kreme doughnuts) that often occurs on the down day simply vanishes on the up day. Over a period of weeks, most people find that they begin to choose healthier foods, especially vegetables. It's unclear exactly why this shift occurs, but it may be that your body's perception of a low energy supply triggers a genetic program that tells you to eat a diet high in nutrients, meaning that you find vegetarian sources more appealing than before. Another possible explanation is that because (after the initial two weeks when you reintroduce regular food) you are hungrier on the down days and choose to eat more vegetables in order to reduce caloric intake subsequently, you find them better-tasting because they may be preferable to other "diet" choices. Whatever the cause, I have noticed a trend to greatly increase vegetable consumption on the up days and—after the initial two weeks—on the down days as well.

9.

Step 2: The Alternate-Day Diet for Life

After two weeks, your SIRT1 gene will be fully activated and working for you. You'll have a better sense of what it means to be hungry, and you'll already have begun to see and feel the benefits of up-day, down-day dieting. You'll have lost some weight and you'll be feeling more energetic. If you have allergies, asthma, or arthritis, you will have started to see a reduction of symptoms.

Now is the time to begin to eat regular food and, depending on how much weight you want to lose, also increase your calorie consumption on your down days. As with most things in life, however, this increased freedom carries with it added risks—in this case the risk that you will begin to rationalize and deceive yourself about how much you're really eating. If you stop losing weight, 98 percent of the time it is because you are taking in too many calories on the down days. I'm not saying that you'll be doing this on purpose, but there is an unconscious tendency within all of us to underestimate the amount we are actually eating.

An Alternate-Day Success Story

My husband has been on the Alternate-Day Diet with me for six months. He was diagnosed as extremely hypertensive (very high blood pressure), with high cholesterol, over twenty years ago and has been on various medications ever since. Seven years ago he had a heart attack. The doctors have always said the same old thing—take the pills, cut fat and sodium, exercise, and lose weight.

Regardless of his weight (which has varied) and his eating/exercise programs (which we worked very hard to get right), his blood pressure was always off the scale. Even with the medication, it refused to come down to a healthy range. He also found it increasingly difficult to lose weight, which may have had something to do with his multiple medications.

One week into this diet his blood pressure was the lowest we have *ever* seen it. Better than that—it was *optimal!* This was also right after treating himself to a burger combo for lunch! Convinced that this must have been some kind of mistake, we have carefully monitored his blood pressure frequently since. He is getting the same consistent low readings. He is now also 20 pounds lighter and much happier. Needless to say, we are delighted. Maybe it's time to discuss cutting meds with the doctor!

—Mrs. G. M.

Keeping that journal we talked about earlier and writing down what you're eating on your down days is a good way to keep this from happening. The point at which you should also start keeping a record of what you're eating on your up days is when you stop losing weight or begin to lose less than a pound a week. The objective is to maintain the sense of freedom alternate-day restriction provides without falling off the wagon, so to speak. Keeping a journal can actually bolster your enthusiasm and help you remain motivated to press onward and downward.

ADJUSTING YOUR DOWN-DAY CALORIES

It stands to reason, of course, that the fewer calories you take in on your down days the better off you'll be, particularly if your goal is to lose weight, not simply to maintain your weight and improve your health. If you switch to eating real food after the initial induction period and can still keep your down-day calorie intake to no more than 20 percent of normal, that would be great—and many people do it without any problem. For others, however, 20 percent feels too restrictive for long-term compliance (which is, obviously, the key to success on any diet). I would suggest that you try it at 20 percent for at least a week and see how you feel. If it's too difficult or unpleasant for you, try going to 25 or 35 percent.

Within this range you can have tasty meals that will leave you satisfied. You won't feel as deprived as you were during the first two weeks of the diet, which means that you'll be more likely to stay with it. My goal here is to be practical. If you feel as deprived as you probably have felt on all the diets you've quit, you won't continue on this one either. I'm therefore recommending as few calories as I believe you'll find tolerable over the long haul.

Personally, although I sometimes go as low as 30 percent, I regularly eat approximately 50 percent of my normal intake on alternate days for a couple of reasons: I know that this level of reduction is enough to activate SIRT1 and give me significant health benefits, and it's the level at which I'm most comfortable and don't gain weight. I would always like to lose a few more pounds, as most of us probably would, but I've been unable to maintain a lower weight over time, so I have decided to stay at the 50 percent level (or lower).

I might be described as a backsliding reformed disinhibitor. Disinhibitors are usually men who like to eat and who describe themselves as "big eaters" in an almost macho sense. Restrainers, by contrast, are typically young women who are concerned about their body weight for reasons of appearance. I have come to realize the danger of being a disinhibitor in the present food environment, but I do have a natural inclination to overeat, and only by restricting my caloric intake every other day can I keep my weight from creeping upward.

Know Yourself and You Will Be Free

I know that many people would prefer to be told exactly what to eat when and how much on every day of a diet, but if you're looking at "diet" as a lifelong lifestyle, rather than an on-again, off-again quick fix, that simply isn't practical. No one is going to stick to such restriction very long—and the proof is that despite the vast number of diets available to everyone, the great majority of us remain overweight.

The Alternate-Day Diet succeeds because it allows you to determine the level of restriction at which you are comfortable and requires you to restrict only on alternate days. Once you determine the level of down-day restriction you can live with (up to 50 percent) and make sure that you stick to that, you'll never again have to worry about "cheating" or eating "bad" food at a party, or never having a cheeseburger again for the rest of your life, because you'll be able to do all of that at least every other day.

Actually, as indicated by the study done by Ravussin and his colleagues that we discussed on page 61, eating 75 percent of required calories every day activates the SIRT1-mediated calorie restriction mechanism, and we believe that this level of restriction for a 36-hour period of lower energy, as provided by the Alternate-Day Diet, is sufficient to turn on SIRT1, although not as intensively as lower intakes on the down day.

It's About Maintaining a Balance

Remember that I'm not advocating *overeating* on your up days, but you do need to eat normally not just to prevent "diet fatigue" but also to prevent your metabolism from slowing down.

In general, three things happen when you lose weight:

- During normal weight loss (if you're dieting every day), after a few days your metabolism slows down by about 15 percent and remains at that level as long as you continue to lose weight.
- Once you've stopped losing weight your metabolism stabilizes, but there is some evidence to suggest that there may be a long-term reduction in metabolic rate of about 3 or 4 percent in the average person.
- Once you weigh less, you will need fewer calories to maintain your weight even if your metabolic rate isn't reduced. This ought to be fairly obvious—if your body weighs less, it consumes fewer calories.

No diet can change the fact that the less you weigh, the less you can eat without gaining weight, but following the Alternate-Day Diet will at least prevent the reduction in metabolic rate that occurs with other diets. Because you're not restricting calories every day, your body doesn't perceive that it is "starving" (which is what triggers calorie conservation through a reduction in metabolic rate), and therefore your metabolism doesn't slow down. This principle was demonstrated in Ravussin's study of volunteers who ate every other day for three weeks. Their resting metabolic rate did not go down. This is one of the great benefits of the Alternate-Day Diet.

Don't Go Overboard

According to anecdotal evidence disseminated by the cruise industry, the average person gains 8 pounds in the course of a seven-day cruise. Based on the average American BMI of 26 or 27, my own calculations indicate that these people must be eating about 250 percent of their normal calorie intake every day throughout the entire cruise.

Although that sounds impossible, it probably isn't, especially when you're being invited to partake of an abundance of good, tasty free food virtually nonstop and you're also on vacation, outside your usual daily routine, and you know it isn't going to last forever. What you should recognize is that you are capable of greatly increasing the amount you eat if you allow yourself to eat without any attempt at self-control.

The moral of this story is that life isn't a cruise, and while I don't advocate that you restrict calories on your up days, I also caution you against throwing caution to the wind and stuffing yourself. Balance is everything—at the dining table as it is in all of life!

It's tempting, when something is working, to want to do it more and better, and in the Asthma Study it did appear that our study subjects were restricting calories to some degree on their up days. You, too, may begin to think that the less you eat on your up days the better off you'll be, but again, it's a question of balance. You don't want to slow down your metabolism and you also don't want to feel deprived every day—that's nothing less than a prescription for noncompliance and, ultimately, diet failure.

That said, however, the fact remains that in order to lose weight we have to use more calories than we are eating. So whether or not there is a change in metabolic rate with this or any diet, we simply have to accept the fact that we have to restrain ourselves sufficiently to lose weight.

FOODS TO FEED YOUR DOWN DAYS

The following lists are neither exhaustive nor definitive, but they'll get you started on the road to down-day success. Any paperback calorie counter or online calorie site will help you to expand into other foods you enjoy.

Nonstarchy Carbohydrates

The following vegetables are nutrient-dense, full of antioxidants, filling (because they contain water and fiber), and very low in calories:

FOOD	AMOUNT	CALORIES
Artichokes, boiled	4 ounces	50
Asparagus, boiled	4 spears	12
Beans: green or wax	1 pound	128
Bok choy, boiled	½ cup	10

Adapted from *Eat, Drink, and Be Healthy* by Walter Willett, MD, with Patrick J. Skerrett.

FOOD	AMOUNT	CALORIES
Broccoli, boiled	½ cup florets	20
Brussels sprouts, boiled	1 cup (7 to 8 sprouts)	56
Cabbage, green	1 cup shredded	18
Carrots, raw	1 cup sliced	52
Cauliflower, boiled	6 florets	25
Eggplant, boiled	½ cup cubes	14
Greens: collard, kale, mustard, or turnip, boiled	½ cup	25
Lettuce: butterhead, Boston, Bibb	1 cup shredded	7
Mushrooms, raw	1 cup whole	24
Okra, boiled	½ cup sliced	26
Pea pods, boiled	½ cup	34
Peppers: green, red, yellow, or orange, raw	1 cup sliced	25
Spinach, boiled	1 cup	36
Squash, boiled	½ cup	15
Tomatoes, raw	1 medium	33
Water chestnuts, canned	½ cup sliced	35
Zucchini, boiled	½ cup sliced	9

Lean Protein

A small amount of protein will help to keep you feeling fuller longer.

Chicken breast		
skinless and boneless, broiled	4 ounces	186
Egg whites	2 large	33
Fish		
Cod	4 ounces cooked	119
Flounder	4 ounces cooked	133
Salmon	4 ounces cooked	233
Snapper	4 ounces cooked	145
Swordfish	4 ounces cooked	145
Tuna	4 ounces cooked	209
Shellfish		
Crab	4 ounces cooked	116
Lobster	4 ounces cooked	111
Shrimp	4 ounces cooked	112
Tofu, silken firm	1 slice	52
Turkey breast		
skinless and boneless, roasted	4 ounces	153

Good Fats

Remember that whether or not they're "healthy," all fats have about 100 calories per tablespoon, so they'll have to be used very sparingly on your down days.

Canola oil
Olive oil
Soybean oil

Down-Day Flavorings and Food Substitutes

Use as many and as much as you like—the more flavorful your food, the more it will satisfy you.

Any dried herbs and spices
Garlic
Ginger, fresh
Hot sauce: Tabasco or Worcestershire
Lemon juice
Low-fat or non-fat broth
No-calorie salad dressings
Nonstick cooking spray
Salt and pepper
Shirataki tofu noodles (see page 189)
Soy sauce (20 calories per tablespoon)
Vinegar: balsamic or wine

Snack Attack

No one's immune, and there will be times when you'll just *have to have* a snack *right now*. Portion control is important when choosing snacks, because a calorie-dense food may be appropriate for a snack when eaten in small amounts but can blow your calories for the day if you eat too much. This is especially true for nuts, nut butters, and cheese. Other foods, such as raw vegetables, are lower in calories and can be eaten in larger amounts. Some companies are now selling 100-calorie packages of foods for snacking.

100 CALORIES OR LESS

3 cups air-popped popcorn

7 walnut halves

10 raw almonds

20 peanuts

25 pistachios

1 cup nonfat milk

1 ounce light string cheese

1 Jell-O nonfat pudding cup

1 hard-cooked large egg (limit if on a
    cholesterol-reduced diet)

1 tablespoon peanut butter

50 CALORIES OR LESS

1 cup chopped raw vegetables

½ cup blueberries or raspberries

½ cup fresh cherries

½ medium banana

3 fresh apricots

1 medium kiwifruit

1 small apple

15 grapes

¾ cup tomato juice

¾ cup vegetable juice cocktail

2 slices melba toast

2 Hershey's Kisses

10 CALORIES OR LESS

½ cup sugar-free gelatin dessert

1 celery stalk

3 cherry tomatoes

1 medium dill pickle

FREE

Coffee, without cream or caloric sweetener

Black or green teas, plain

Diet sodas

DOWN-DAY STRATEGIES FOR
STAYING ON TRACK

Once you've completed the induction phase and are using meal-replacement shakes as your main source of calories on down days, you'll be looking for ways to get through down days with more than just the anticipation of tomorrow.

- Make one of your meals a shake. This will give you one less meal to think about. It's easy, and if you have a shake for breakfast, you'll know exactly how many calories you have to last you the rest of the day. Or if you generally eat lunch on the run, take your shake with you so that you won't be tempted to grab whatever is handy or stop in at your favorite fast-food emporium.
- Eat lean protein. You'll be more satisfied with less. It will keep you feeling fuller longer. And you won't be spiking your blood sugar and triggering cravings for sweets as you will with carbohydrates.
- Keep your measuring implements handy so that you don't underestimate what you're consuming or become tempted to add just one more dab of peanut butter to your cracker.
- Take some physical action to record your calorie intake, such as writing down every time you eat something. This action uses a principle of behavior modification that says "the hand teaches the heart"; that is, the physical action somehow breaks through the denial to which we are all subject. If you cannot commit yourself to writing it down, you are likely to fail.
- Exercise: Intense or prolonged physical activity can affect

An Alternate-Day Cautionary Tale

I've been doing this diet for more than six months and have lost 26 pounds. I have another 23 to lose to reach my goal.

It's still working for me, though the loss does slow down somewhat (like most diets, really). Overall, I have averaged a steady (and very healthy) 1 pound per week. This includes some "mistakes" and a five-week vacation of free eating, which only resulted in a 5-pound gain that amazingly fell off within two weeks of getting back in the game!

As you progress, it's important to check back with the Calorie Calculator (to calculate an estimate of calorie requirements for "down" days) and adjust calories for your lower weight accordingly. After being on this plan for a while, it does become necessary to watch up-day calories too. Though that seems less of an issue, as I just don't *want* large amounts of food anymore. My latest strategy has been to incorporate some of my down-day tricks on up days in order to get the most out of my calorie allowance.

All I can say is that this is *the* easiest diet to stay with. Isn't that the key? If I can do it, anyone can!

I don't see this as a "diet," I see it as a lifestyle, and don't doubt that I will continue to use this forever if I am to maintain my weight when I get there.

—Mrs. J. S.

your down-day calorie requirement. For example, slow jogging for one mile (which takes most people about 20 minutes) burns about 100 calories, allowing you to add

100 calories to your down-day intake. Just be aware that you need to be very honest with yourself about how many extra calories you are burning. Therefore, if it takes you less than 20 minutes, or you don't walk a full mile, don't even count it.

10.

Give Yourself a Break:
An Alternative to Dieting
Every Other Day

As I've said from the beginning, one reason so many people have been willing and able to stick with the Alternate-Day Diet is that they don't have to diet every day. It's about *intermittent* (as opposed to continuous) calorie restriction.

But again, we humans—because we're human—tend to get bored, cheat, or let things slide when we're doing the same thing over a long period of time. Therefore, what I propose is that, if you find that your down-day calorie intake is slowly creeping up, you're skipping a down day here and there, or you're just getting bored, you give yourself a break from the routine by using a different form of intermittent restriction—eating according to your natural circadian rhythm.

Virtually all living things have an innate circadian clock that determines how and when various genes and chemicals in the body are activated and interact with one another. We humans are innately diurnal, meaning that our normal circadian pattern is to be active during the day and sleep at night. Our ancestors lived in accordance with this rhythm because they didn't really have much choice—no artificial light, no late-night TV for entertainment, and the necessity to hunt and gather food when they could see what they were doing. Now, of course, we can, and often do, turn night into day at will. But studies are beginning to indicate that this man-made disruption of our circadian rhythm may not be the healthiest way to live.

In addition to the central clock in our brains, we also have ancillary "time-keepers" in other types of cells that regulate the rise and fall of gene activity throughout a twenty-four-hour cycle. When that cycle is disrupted, we may experience a variety of metabolic dysfunctions that can cause obesity and disease.

Observational studies have shown an increase in breast cancer among night-shift workers. Changes in glucose metabolism that are associated with obesity and diabetes have been shown with a disruption of the circadian clock among pilots, and longtime exposure to artificial light has been linked to an increase in depression that can be remediated with the return to a normal circadian rhythm. The underlying reasons for these changes have not been clearly established, but there seem to be some pretty clear implications to be drawn from these observations.

Melatonin, for example, is a hormone secreted by the pineal gland that is normally released when light decreases—that is, at night. We know that increased melatonin is associated with getting a good night's sleep, but it now appears that the proper release of melatonin at the appropriate time may also be related to other chemical processes in the body that reduce a woman's risk for breast cancer. In fact, several studies have shown an association between increased melatonin levels and a reduction in tumor growth. Melatonin levels decrease in the absence of sleep at night and do not reach optimal growth even when the person is asleep during the day.

In addition, levels of ghrelin, the hormone associated with hunger, have been shown to go down in animals that are fed during a restricted period of time. To me, this is a significant finding because I, and others who have followed the circadian eating pattern, have experienced a reduction in appetite, particularly in the evening.

Also, many people with obesity-related Type 2 diabetes find that their diabetes goes away after gastric bypass surgery, and this may possibly be because many of the cells in the stomach and small intestine that produce ghrelin have been removed, thus reducing their hunger.

In a 2012 study published in the journal *Cell Metabolism*, Dr. Satchidananda Panda and his colleagues compared a group of mice on a high-fat diet who were fed only for an eight-hour period with another group fed an equal number of calories but given free access to their food. The mice on the time-restricted diet were shown to be protected against obesity, hyperinsulinemia, fatty liver, and inflammation and had improved motor coordination. The researchers concluded that a time-restricted feeding regimen was "a non-pharmacological strategy against obesity and associated diseases."

Another study done by Drs. Oren Froy and Ruth Miskin also concluded that "circadian disruption is associated with multiple negative manifestations, whereas resetting of circadian rhythms could lead to increased longevity."

And in February 2013, researchers at Vanderbilt University published a study in *Current Biology* showing that disruption of the body's circadian rhythm can lead not only to obesity but also to an increased risk of diabetes and heart disease resulting from changes in insulin activity. "The master clock in the central nervous system drives the cycle and insulin response follows," says Vanderbilt professor of molecular physiology Owen McGuinness. To prove their hypothesis the researchers removed one of the genes necessary for proper functioning of the biological clock in one group of mice, and found that they appeared to be locked in an insulin-resistant mode. Supplying them with the protein produced by the missing gene reestablished their circadian rhythm and reduced their insulin resistance.

In addition, they kept a group of normal mice in a constantly lit environment that also disrupted their circadian cycle (because mice, unlike humans, are nocturnal and therefore would normally eat at night) and found that this group was locked into an inactive or fasting phase during which they were naturally more insulin resistant and therefore developed a higher proportion of body fat and gained more weight on a high-fat diet than those whose circadian cycle was not artificially disrupted.

Exposure to artificial light disrupts normal circadian rhythms by reducing melatonin production, but not all artificial light is created equal, and it seems that the most harmful is blue light. An article published in the *Harvard Health Letter* in May 2012 states that, "While light of any kind can suppress the secretion of melatonin, blue light does so more powerfully. Harvard researchers and their colleagues conducted an experiment comparing the effects of 6.5 hours of exposure to blue light to exposure to green light of comparable brightness. The blue light suppressed melatonin for about twice as long as the green light and shifted circadian rhythms by twice as much (3 hours vs. 1.5 hours)."

While in the modern world it would be difficult to avoid artificial light entirely, we can minimize our exposure to the dangers of blue light by putting filters on our computer screens and wearing glasses that block only blue light without blocking other colors as inexpensive sunglasses do. Personally, I usually wear blue-light blocking amber glasses after eight or nine o'clock at night. I do this because I believe that this simple measure will help to increase melatonin levels, which will, in turn, help to prevent disease as well as to ameliorate diseases I might already have.

So, getting back to "giving yourself a break" by following a circadian pattern of intermittent calorie restriction, my point is that there's more than one way to skin a cat, so to speak. Eating all your meals during an eight-hour period during the day means that you will be fasting for sixteen hours during every twenty-four-hour period. You will not only be reaping the benefits of calorie cycling without any overall reduction in your intake but you will also be accruing the health benefits derived from maintaining a robust pattern of metabolic gene expression.

My suggestion would be that if or when you feel that you need a break from the Alternate-Day Diet, you switch to the circadian pattern for a period of three weeks. During that time you can eat as much as you normally would but your entire caloric intake must be within a period of eight hours. That will probably mean skipping or delaying your breakfast and having your dinner before eight o'clock at night. The most important thing is to follow the pattern, do the same thing every day, and avoid disrupting your melatonin production by limiting your exposure to artificial blue light.

While restricting calories on your down day is the most difficult aspect of sticking to the Alternate-Day Diet, eating within this confined period of time is the challenge for most people on the circadian eating plan.

After three weeks of following the circadian plan you will probably find that you have actually lost some weight even though you have not reduced your caloric intake. I suggest that at this point you return to the alternate-day pattern, eating 30 to 50 percent of normal on the down day, which is less of a restriction than is typically suggested but will make it easier to stick to the pattern over time.

You can continue to switch from one to the other, thereby keeping yourself motivated, interested, healthy, and slim for life.

11.

Delicious Down-Day
Menus and Recipes

Once you've completed the initial two-week period when you're using meal-replacement shakes on your down days, you'll probably want to know what you can eat to vary meals on your down days and still feel satisfied. The following recipes are designed to help you do just that.

The recipes in this chapter are easy to prepare and, in general, use ingredients that are readily available. You will notice that most of the main dishes include fish or chicken and turkey white meat, although there are also some vegetarian entrées. That's because these foods usually have lower amounts of fat, especially saturated fat, and calories than beef, or turkey and chicken legs and thighs (the dark meat). Salmon and darker-fleshed fish are generally higher in fat and have a more pronounced flavor than white fish, but they are also higher in the good fats, such as the omega-3 fatty acids that promote heart health.

When fats are reduced in cooking, it is important to add herbs, spices, fresh lemon juice, and other flavor-enhancing ingredients to make the recipes flavorful enough that you won't miss the fat.

Many of the down-day recipes would also be excellent choices for the up days—just increase the portion size, add an extra serving of vegetables, add a side dish of noodles or rice, or add a whole-grain, artisan-style bread. You could also add a dessert or a glass of wine to your dinner to make it an up-day meal.

STOCK YOUR DOWN-DAY LARDER

It will be easier to watch calories on your down days if you have everything you need on hand. That way you'll have no excuse for cheating because "it's all I had in the kitchen." And, of course, the same foods can also be used to prepare up-day meals.

PANTRY
Beans: canned, dried; regular and low-sodium
Cereals: high-fiber, low-sugar
Chicken broth: low-sodium
Flavoring extracts
Herbs and spices, dried
Meal-replacement drinks
Oatmeal: old fashioned
Olive oil: extra-virgin
Olive oil cooking spray
Peanut butter: natural with no added salt or sugar
Popcorn for air-popping
Salad dressing: low-fat, such as Newman's Own
Tomatoes: canned

Vegetable juices: preferably low-sodium
Whole-grain products: bread, pasta, and brown rice

REFRIGERATOR

Cheeses: low-fat
Egg substitute
Fruits and vegetables
Herbs: fresh
Milk: nonfat
Salad greens and other salad ingredients
Shirataki tofu noodles (see page 189)
Tofu
Yogurt: nonfat

FREEZER

Chicken breasts: preferably individually wrapped
Fish: preferably individually wrapped
Fruits: unsweetened
Shrimp: raw, unbreaded
Vegetables: plain, without added butter or sauces

EQUIP YOUR KITCHEN

Most of the recipes in this book are very easy to prepare and require no special equipment, but there are a few items that will make it easier to prepare your meals, especially low-calorie ones.

Blender: A blender is needed to make smoothies and other drinks. It can also be used to chop nuts and make bread crumbs.

Collapsible steamer rack: This inexpensive but helpful utensil turns any pot into a steamer for vegetables.

Food processor: Essential for preparing many soups, especially ones that are thickened by pureeing some of the ingredients rather than using cream. Food processors are also great for blending ingredients for sauces and dips, chopping meats, and preparing dough.

Kitchen scale: A scale makes portion control easy, especially for items such as meats, nuts, and cheeses.

Measuring cups: You'll need both liquid and dry measures, not only to ensure that you're using the correct proportions of ingredients but also to keep yourself honest in terms of the quantity you're eating on your down days.

Measuring spoons: As with measuring cups, these are important to make sure that you're following the recipes accurately.

Nonstick cookware: If you use nonstick pots and pans, you can sauté vegetables or meats simply by spraying the pan with a little cooking spray rather than using oil or butter, which add calories and fat. The foods will not stick to the pan, and cleanup is quick and easy.

Plastic or wooden spatulas and large spoons: Use these instead of metal ones to keep your nonstick cookware scratch-free.

Salad spinner: Makes washing and drying salad greens a snap. A salad spinner is the secret to crisp salads.

The Menus

Since the following menus are only for your down days (the up days are up to you), they will keep you on track for a full 30 days. But even on the down days, you have options:

- Substitute a meal-replacement shake for one of the meals.
- Depending on your schedule, you can switch the lunch and dinner menus.
- There are a few low-calorie snacks that can be added to the menus as needed. In addition, if you want something to munch on, it's a great idea to keep raw vegetables, such as celery and carrot sticks, cucumber and jicama slices, radishes, and cherry tomatoes in the refrigerator. (For further down-day snack ideas, see page 141).
- If the menu does not include a salad, one cup of mixed greens with a low-fat dressing, such as Newman's Own, will add less than 50 calories to your meal.

Day 1: Down Day

BREAKFAST

Creamy Oats and Berries
(page 172)
Calories: 191

LUNCH

Tomato and Roasted Bell Pepper
Soup (page 181)
Calories: 159

DINNER

Roasted Salmon, Asparagus, Bell
Pepper, and Mushrooms
(page 208)
Calories: 248

TOTAL CALORIES: 598

Day 2: Up Day

Your choice

Day 3: Down Day

BREAKFAST

1 slice high-fiber, whole-grain
bread, toasted
1 tablespoon peanut butter
Calories: 154

LUNCH

Asian Chicken Noodle Soup
(page 187)
Calories: 165

DINNER

Turkey and White Bean Chili
(page 220)
Calories: 210

TOTAL CALORIES: 529

Day 4: Up Day

Your choice

Day 5: Down Day

BREAKFAST

1 cup Kashi 7 whole-grain flakes

1/2 cup nonfat milk

Calories: 225

LUNCH

Egg Drop Soup (page 186)

Calories: 91

Mixed Greens Tossed with
    Noodles (page 200)

Calories: 100

DINNER

Trout with Capers and Lemon
    (page 206)

1 cup broccoli

Calories: 260

TOTAL CALORIES: 676

Day 6: Up Day

Your choice

Day 7: Down Day

BREAKFAST

Broccoli Frittata (page 169)

Calories: 126

LUNCH

Mixed Seafood in Tomato Broth
    (page 184)

Calories: 231

DINNER

Sesame-Crusted Baked Chicken
    Breasts on Napa Cabbage
    (page 214)

Calories: 289

TOTAL CALORIES: 646

Day 8: Up Day

Your choice

Day 9: Down Day

BREAKFAST
Strawberry-Yogurt Smoothie
(page 170)
Calories: 234

LUNCH
Vietnamese Soup (page 188)
Calories: 206

DINNER
Broiled Halibut and Cherry
Tomatoes Florentine
(page 203)
Calories: 159

TOTAL CALORIES: 599

Day 10: Up Day
Your choice

Day 11: Down Day

BREAKFAST
½ slice high-fiber, whole-grain
English muffin, toasted
1 tablespoon peanut butter
Calories: 159

LUNCH
Diced Apple and Tuna Salad
with Lettuce and Cucumber
Wedges (page 196)
Calories: 165

SNACK
Goat Cheese–Stuffed Endive
with Fresh Tomatoes
(page 176)
Calories: 47

DINNER
Chicken with Artichoke Hearts
Italiano (page 211)
Calories: 217

TOTAL CALORIES: 588

Day 12: Up Day
Your choice

Day 13: Down Day

BREAKFAST
2/3 cup cooked oatmeal
1/2 cup nonfat milk
Calories: 154

LUNCH
Asparagus, Carrot, and Peas
    in Broth (page 185)
Calories: 148
Watermelon and Tomato Salad
    with Goat Cheese
    (page 191)
Calories: 126

DINNER
Seared Scallops in Tarragon
    Sauce (page 210)
1 cup green beans
Calories: 225

TOTAL CALORIES: 653

Day 14: Up Day
Your choice

Day 15: Down Day

BREAKFAST
1/2 cup high-fiber cereal, such
    as Fiber One or All-Bran
1/2 cup nonfat milk
Calories: 100

LUNCH
White Bean–Artichoke Heart
    Salad (page 193)
Calories: 276

DINNER
Grilled Pork Tenderloin, Onion,
    and Bell Peppers (page 221)
Calories: 173

TOTAL CALORIES: 549

Day 16: Up Day
Your choice

Day 17: Down Day

BREAKFAST

Banana-Raspberry Smoothie
    (page 171)

Calories: 220

LUNCH

Crab Cakes on Greens with
    Green Beans and Tomatoes
    (page 201)

Calories: 237

DINNER

Roasted Turkey Meatballs in
    Creamy Yogurt Sauce
    (page 216)

1 cup sugar snap peas

Calories: 231

TOTAL CALORIES: 688

Day 18: Up Day

Your choice

Day 19: Down Day

BREAKFAST

2/3 cup cooked oatmeal

1/2 cup nonfat milk

Calories: 154

LUNCH

White Bean and Greens Soup
    (page 179)

Calories: 184

Spinach-Couscous Salad
    (page 199)

Calories: 118

DINNER

Turkey Cutlets with Thyme-
    Mustard Sauce (page 217)

Calories: 166

TOTAL CALORIES: 622

Day 20: Up Day

Your choice

Day 21: Down Day

BREAKFAST
½ cup high-fiber cereal, such
    as Fiber One or All-Bran
½ cup nonfat milk
Calories: 100

LUNCH
Caribbean Black Bean Soup
    (page 183)
Calories: 265
Jicama, Orange, and Arugula
    Salad (page 198)
Calories: 114

DINNER
Vegetable-Topped Fish in the
    Microwave, Mexican-Style
    (page 209)
Calories: 176

TOTAL CALORIES: 655

Day 22: Up Day
Your choice

Day 23: Down Day

BREAKFAST
⅔ cup cooked oatmeal
½ cup nonfat milk
Calories: 154

LUNCH
Creamy Cauliflower Soup
    (page 178)
Calories: 191

DINNER
Chicken with Pineapple, Bell
    Peppers, and Onions
    (page 213)
Calories: 236

TOTAL CALORIES: 581

Day 24: Up Day
Your choice

Day 25: Down Day

BREAKFAST
Blueberry-Tofu Smoothie
(page 170)
Calories: 240

LUNCH
Italian Summer Squash Soup
(page 182)
Calories: 113
Romaine Hearts with Buttermilk
Dressing (page 194)
Calories: 73

DINNER
Grilled Fish with Papaya–Bell
Pepper Salsa (page 207)
Calories: 182

TOTAL CALORIES: 608

Day 26: Up Day
Your choice

Day 27: Down Day

BREAKFAST
1 cup Kashi 7 whole-grain flakes
½ cup nonfat milk
Calories: 225

LUNCH
Creamy Broccoli-Cheese Soup
(page 180)
Calories: 212

DINNER
Shredded Chicken and
Vegetables in Lettuce Leaf
Cups (page 212)
Calories: 174

TOTAL CALORIES: 611

Day 28: Up Day
Your choice

Day 29: Down Day

BREAKFAST

Vegetable Omelet (page 168)

Calories: 128

1 slice high-fiber, whole-grain
   bread

Calories: 60

LUNCH

Garbanzo Bean–Spinach Salad
   (page 192)

Calories: 183

DINNER

Soft Fish Tacos (page 205)

Calories: 296

TOTAL CALORIES: 667

Day 30: Up Day

Your choice

The Recipes

Breakfasts and Snacks

Soups

Salads

Main Dishes

About the Nutritional Analysis

All the recipes were analyzed using the Food Processor, Version 8.1, software program. Any ingredients that are to taste, such as salt and pepper, or are optional are not included in the analysis. When there is a choice of ingredients in a recipe, the first ingredient is used for the analysis. When a recipe yield is a range, such as 2 or 3 servings or 4 to 6 servings, the first number is used, and if you divide the recipe into the larger number of servings, the calorie count and other values will be slightly less.

VEGETABLE OMELET

Makes 2 servings

If you don't want to have this for breakfast, try it at lunchtime instead. Or make it a light supper.

½ cup chopped fresh
  mushrooms
½ cup chopped green bell
  pepper

Salt and freshly ground black
  pepper, to taste
1 cup egg substitute
1 Roma tomato, diced

Spray a medium nonstick skillet with cooking spray and heat over medium heat. Add the mushrooms and bell pepper and cook, stirring occasionally, until softened, about 5 minutes. Season with salt and black pepper, transfer to a bowl, and wipe out the skillet with a damp paper towel.

Spray the skillet again with cooking spray and heat over medium heat. Add the egg substitute and cook until the center starts to set, about 2 minutes. Spoon the vegetables over the omelet. Lift with a spatula so the uncooked portion of egg can flow to the edge to cook. Cut the omelet in half, transfer to two plates, and top each serving with diced tomato.

Per serving: Calories 128, Protein 16g, Total fat 4g, Sat fat 1g, Trans fat 0g,
Cholesterol 1mg, Carbohydrate 6g, Dietary fiber 1g, Sodium 227mg

BROCCOLI FRITTATA

Makes 2 servings

Frittatas are similar to omelets except they are usually thicker and either finished under the broiler or turned onto a plate and returned to the skillet uncooked side down.

1 cup broccoli florets, cut into bite-size pieces

½ cup chopped red bell pepper

2 tablespoons chopped fresh chives or green onion tops

1 cup egg substitute

Dash of hot pepper sauce

Freshly ground black pepper, to taste

Bring a pot of water to a boil. Add the broccoli and bring back to a boil. Add the bell pepper. Drain and cool under cold running water.

Preheat the broiler. Combine the vegetables, chives, and egg substitute in a bowl. Season with the hot pepper sauce and black pepper. Spray a small nonstick skillet with a heatproof handle with cooking spray and heat over medium heat. Add the vegetable mixture and cook until the egg substitute begins to set, about 4 minutes.

Place the skillet under the broiler and cook until the top of the mixture is set, about 3 minutes. Watch carefully to prevent burning, because the time may vary. Cut the frittata in half and transfer to two plates.

Per serving: Calories 126, Protein 17g, Total fat 4g, Sat fat 1g, Trans fat 0g, Cholesterol 1mg, Carbohydrate 5g, Dietary fiber 2g, Sodium 232mg

STRAWBERRY-YOGURT SMOOTHIE

Makes about 2½ cups

◇◇

If the strawberries are sweet and ripe, you will not need any additional sweetener. If you like it sweeter, add 1 teaspoon honey (20 calories).

1 cup chopped fresh or frozen
  strawberries

½ cup plain nonfat yogurt
1 cup nonfat milk

Combine all the ingredients in a blender and process until smooth.

Per recipe: Calories 234, Protein 15g, Total fat 1g, Sat fat 0.4g, Trans fat 0g, Cholesterol 6mg, Carbohydrate 42g, Dietary fiber 3g, Sodium 205mg

BLUEBERRY-TOFU SMOOTHIE

Makes about 2½ cups

◇◇

Using frozen fruit will make the smoothie thicker. Add more milk if needed to reach the desired consistency—each additional tablespoon of nonfat milk will add about 5 calories.

½ cup silken tofu
1 cup fresh or frozen
  blueberries

½ cup nonfat milk or soy milk
  (see Note)
½ cup orange juice

Combine all the ingredients in a blender in the order listed and process until smooth.

Per recipe: Calories 240, Protein 11g, Total fat 4g, Sat fat 0.7g, Trans fat 0g, Cholesterol 2mg, Carbohydrate 41g, Dietary fiber 4g, Sodium 71mg

Note: *Nonfat, fat-free, and skim milk are all milk that has had the fat removed. Nonfat milk is still an excellent source of calcium and vitamin D.*

BANANA-RASPBERRY SMOOTHIE

Makes about 2 cups

When using soy protein powder, adding banana makes a smoother-textured drink.

½ medium banana, chopped

½ cup fresh or frozen raspberries

1 cup nonfat milk or soy milk

2 tablespoons soy protein powder

¼ teaspoon vanilla extract

Combine the banana and raspberries in a blender. Top with the milk, protein powder, and vanilla and process until smooth.

Per recipe: Calories 220, Protein 22g, Total fat 1g, Sat fat 0.4g, Trans fat 0g, Cholesterol 5mg, Carbohydrate 32g, Dietary fiber 3g, Sodium 274mg

CREAMY OATS AND
BERRIES

Makes 1 serving

This crunchy, sweet parfait will make you think you're eating dessert for breakfast

2 tablespoons old-fashioned rolled
  oats

½ cup plain nonfat yogurt

1 tablespoon maple syrup, rice
  syrup, or other sweetener of
  choice

1 teaspoon vanilla extract or
  ½ teaspoon ground cinnamon

½ cup blueberries, blackberries,
  or strawberries, or a
  combination

Toast the oats in a small heavy skillet over medium heat, stirring constantly, until lightly browned. Let cool to room temperature.

Combine the yogurt, maple syrup, and vanilla in a small bowl. Stir in the oats. Spoon half of the yogurt mixture into a glass dish and top with half of the berries. Repeat the layers.

Per serving: Calories 191, Protein 7g, Total fat 1g, Sat fat 0g, Trans fat 0g, Cholesterol 2mg, Carbohydrate 40g, Dietary fiber 3g, Sodium 74mg

LEMONY HUMMUS

Makes 6 servings; about 1½ cups

Use this to dip baby carrots, broccoli or cauliflower florets, or any vegetable of your choice. It will keep, tightly covered, in the refrigerator for up to 3 days.

1 (15-ounce) can garbanzo beans, rinsed and drained

3 tablespoons freshly squeezed lemon juice

1 tablespoon freshly grated lemon zest

2 large garlic cloves, minced

1 tablespoon toasted sesame oil

½ teaspoon ground cumin

½ teaspoon ground chipotle chile

½ teaspoon ground coriander

¼ cup plain nonfat yogurt

Combine all the ingredients in a food processor and process until smooth. Transfer to a small bowl, cover, and refrigerate for 30 minutes or overnight for flavors to blend.

Per ¼ cup: Calories 84, Protein 4g, Total fat 3g, Sat fat 0g, Trans fat 0g, Cholesterol 0mg, Carbohydrate 11g, Dietary fiber 3g, Sodium 193mg

PINK SALMON SPREAD

Makes 1 cup

Wild salmon contains more of the omega-3 fatty acids that are important for heart health than farmed salmon, and it is more environmentally friendly.

1 (6-ounce) can pink salmon, preferably wild

1 tablespoon pickle relish, drained

¼ cup minced celery

3 tablespoons plain nonfat yogurt

1 teaspoon freshly squeezed lemon juice

¼ teaspoon dried dillweed (optional)

Combine all the ingredients in a medium bowl and beat until well combined. Use this to fill celery stalks, as a dip, or as a spread on whole-wheat crackers. It will keep, tightly covered, in the refrigerator for up to 3 days.

Per 2 tablespoons: Calories 35, Protein 4g, Total fat 1g, Sat fat 0.3g, Trans fat 0g, Cholesterol 12mg, Carbohydrate 1g, Dietary fiber 0g, Sodium 140mg

HERBED SUN-DRIED TOMATO YOGURT DIP

Makes about 1 cup

Use as a spread on whole-wheat crackers or as a dip for raw vegetables. It will keep, tightly covered, in the refrigerator for up to 3 days.

Packages of soft sun-dried tomatoes are available in the produce section of most supermarkets. They are superior to the harder dried version. They should be refrigerated after opening.

2 tablespoons coarsely chopped, soft sun-dried tomatoes (not oil-packed)

1 cup plain nonfat Greek yogurt or drained yogurt (see Note)

2 tablespoons minced fresh herbs, such as parsley, basil, mint, cilantro, or chives, or a combination

Dash of hot pepper sauce

Put the tomatoes in a food processor and process until finely chopped. Add the yogurt and process until combined. Transfer to a small bowl and stir in the herbs and hot pepper sauce.

Per ¼ cup: Calories 30, Protein 3g, Total fat 0g, Sat fat 0g, Trans fat 0g, Cholesterol 1mg, Carbohydrate 6g, Dietary fiber 0g, Sodium 70mg

Note: *To drain yogurt, spoon 2 cups plain nonfat yogurt without gelatin or other stabilizers into a strainer lined with a coffee filter. Set over a bowl and refrigerate overnight. Discard the liquid. Makes 1 cup.*

GOAT CHEESE-STUFFED ENDIVE WITH FRESH TOMATOES

Makes 1 serving

◇◇

This makes a great hors d'oeuvre even if you're not on the down day of your diet.

3 Belgian endive leaves

2 tablespoons soft low-fat goat cheese (see Note)

1 tablespoon plain nonfat yogurt

Freshly ground black pepper, to taste

2 tablespoons diced fresh tomato

1 tablespoon shredded fresh basil

Rinse the endive thoroughly and dry well. Combine the goat cheese and yogurt in a small bowl. Season with pepper. Divide cheese mixture among the endive leaves and arrange on a plate. Top with the tomato and basil.

Per serving: Calories 47, Protein 2g, Total fat 6g, Sat fat 1g, Trans fat 0g, Cholesterol 10mg, Carbohydrate 4g, Dietary fiber 1g, Sodium 100mg

Note: *Look for low-fat goat cheese in well-stocked supermarkets and specialty stores. Trader Joe's has an excellent one—full of tangy flavor. You won't miss the fat.*

MELON REFRESCA

Makes 1 serving

The small amount of coconut juice in this recipe adds a creamy flavor and only about 20 calories.

1 cup chopped cantaloupe or other melon

1/2 cup crushed ice

1/4 teaspoon grated fresh ginger, or to taste

1/4 cup coconut juice with pulp (see Note)

Combine all the ingredients in a blender and puree.

Per serving: Calories 77, Protein 1g, Total fat 0.4g, Sat fat 0g, Trans fat 0g, Cholesterol 0mg, Carbohydrate 18g, Dietary fiber 1g, Sodium 31mg

Note: *Coconut juice is the low-fat liquid, usually containing bits of soft pulp, found inside a green or young coconut. It is different from the coconut milk made from mature coconut pulp. You can find canned coconut juice in Latino markets and natural food stores. If unavailable, substitute an equal quantity of water and a dash of coconut extract.*

CREAMY CAULIFLOWER
SOUP

Makes 2 servings; about 2½ cups

You'll be amazed how much rich and creamy texture the nonfat milk in this recipe will provide.

½ cup chopped onion

½ small head cauliflower, broken
into florets

1 (14-ounce) can reduced-sodium
chicken broth

½ cup nonfat milk

Salt and white pepper, to taste

Freshly grated nutmeg, to taste

Chopped fresh chives, for garnish

Combine the onion, cauliflower, and broth in a medium saucepan. Bring to a boil over medium heat. Reduce heat to low, cover, and simmer until cauliflower is tender, for about 15 minutes.

Transfer the soup to a food processor and puree. Return to the saucepan and add the milk. Heat until hot and season with salt, white pepper, and nutmeg. Ladle into two bowls and top with chives.

Per serving: Calories 191, Protein 16g, Total fat 4g, Sat fat 2g, Trans fat 0g, Cholesterol 5mg, Carbohydrate 28g, Dietary fiber 7g, Sodium 166mg

White Bean and
Greens Soup
Makes 4 servings; about 5 cups

The key to using cheese in low-fat cooking is to choose a full-flavored cheese such as Parmesan, which adds a burst of flavor even when used in small amounts. But don't even think about the commercially processed stuff; buy the freshly grated cheese in plastic containers found in the supermarket's cheese case—or better yet, buy a wedge and grate it yourself.

1 large garlic clove, minced

1 shallot, minced

2 cups frozen chopped greens (turnip greens, mustard greens, collards, or spinach)

3 cups reduced-sodium chicken broth

1 (15-ounce) can white beans, such as cannellini, navy beans, or butter beans, drained and rinsed

1 teaspoon chopped fresh savory or ½ teaspoon dried

Salt and freshly ground black pepper, to taste

4 tablespoons freshly grated Parmesan cheese, for garnish

Spray a large saucepan with cooking spray. Add the garlic and shallot and cook over medium heat, stirring, until softened. Add the greens and broth. Bring to a boil. Reduce the heat, cover, and simmer until the greens are tender, about 15 minutes. Add the beans and savory and season with salt and pepper. Simmer for about 10 minutes to combine flavors. Ladle into four soup bowls and top each serving with 1 tablespoon of the Parmesan cheese.

Per serving: Calories 184, Protein 13g, Total fat 3g, Sat fat 2g, Trans fat 0g, Cholesterol 7mg, Carbohydrate 27g, Dietary fiber 6g, Sodium 188mg

CREAMY BROCCOLI-
CHEESE SOUP

Makes 2 servings; about 3 cups

*Broccoli is low in calories and high in health-protecting antioxi-
dants, but you'll love it just because it's delicious.*

½ cup chopped onion

1 cup fresh or frozen broccoli florets
   (about 8 ounces)

1 small potato (about 4 ounces),
   peeled and cubed

½ cup reduced-sodium chicken
   broth

2 ounces reduced-fat cheese, such
   as cheddar or Mexican blend

Salt and freshly ground black
   pepper, to taste

Dash of hot pepper sauce

Combine the onion, broccoli, potato, and broth in a medium saucepan. Bring to a boil over medium heat. Reduce the heat to low, cover, and simmer until the broccoli is tender, about 15 minutes.

Transfer the soup to a food processor and process until finely chopped but not pureed. Return to the saucepan and add the cheese. Heat, stirring, until the cheese melts. Season with salt and pepper, and stir in a dash of hot pepper sauce. Ladle into two bowls and serve.

Per serving: Calories 212, Protein 16g, Total fat 9g, Sat fat 5g, Trans fat 0g,
Cholesterol 27mg, Carbohydrate 22g, Dietary fiber 5g, Sodium 186mg

TOMATO AND ROASTED BELL PEPPER SOUP

Makes 3 servings; about 4½ cups

Cooking tomatoes allows you to reap the benefits of the powerful antioxidant lycopene that isn't readily absorbed in the body when they're raw. The fresh basil gives even canned tomatoes a fresh-from-the-garden taste.

½ cup chopped onion

1 garlic clove, minced

2 (14-ounce) cans reduced-sodium chicken broth

1 (14.5-ounce) can diced tomatoes with juice

1 (12-ounce) jar roasted bell peppers, drained and rinsed

2 tablespoons finely chopped fresh basil, plus additional for garnish

Freshly ground black pepper, to taste

2 ounces reduced-fat or nonfat cream cheese

Combine the onion, the garlic, and ½ cup of the broth in a medium saucepan over medium heat. Cook, stirring occasionally, until the broth evaporates and the onion starts to caramelize. (Do not burn or the onion will have a bitter flavor.) Add the remaining broth, the tomatoes, and the bell peppers. Simmer, covered, for about 10 minutes for flavors to blend. Remove from heat and stir in the basil. Season with black pepper.

Transfer half the soup to a food processor and add half the cream cheese. Process until still slightly chunky; do not puree. Repeat with the remaining soup and cheese. Reheat, ladle into three bowls, and garnish with the additional basil.

Per serving: Calories 159, Protein 7g, Total fat 5g, Sat fat 3g, Trans fat 0g, Cholesterol 15mg, Carbohydrate 24g, Dietary fiber 3g, Sodium 579mg

Soup

ITALIAN SUMMER
SQUASH SOUP

Makes 3 servings; about 5½ cups

Who would believe anything so easy could be so tasty—and so low in calories!

1 large yellow summer squash (about 8 ounces), chopped

1 medium zucchini (about 8 ounces), chopped

1 celery stalk, finely chopped

½ cup chopped onion

2 garlic cloves, minced

1 (14-ounce) can reduced-sodium chicken broth

1 (14.5-ounce) can diced tomatoes with juice

1 teaspoon chopped fresh oregano or ½ teaspoon dried

2 teaspoons chopped fresh basil or 1 teaspoon dried

Salt and freshly ground black pepper, to taste

3 tablespoons freshly grated Parmesan cheese

Combine all the ingredients except the cheese in a medium saucepan over medium heat. Bring to a boil. Reduce the heat, cover, and simmer until the vegetables are tender, about 15 minutes.

Transfer about 2 cups of the soup to a food processor and process until almost smooth. Return the processed soup to the soup remaining in the pan and heat until hot. Ladle into three bowls and top each serving with 1 tablespoon of the Parmesan cheese.

Per serving: Calories 113, Protein 8g, Total fat 3g, Sat fat 1g, Trans fat 0g, Cholesterol 6mg, Carbohydrate 15g, Dietary fiber 5g, Sodium 358mg

CARIBBEAN BLACK BEAN SOUP

Makes 3 servings; about 3½ cups

Fiber, folate, and antioxidants called anthocyanins mean that black beans are among the healthiest of food choices you can make. Take care when you're mincing the jalapeño not to rub your eyes—the oils in the chile can really make them sting.

2 (15-ounce) cans black beans, drained and rinsed

1 (14-ounce) can reduced-sodium chicken broth

Pinch of dried thyme

1 bay leaf

Dash of hot pepper sauce, or to taste

3 tablespoons chopped tomato

3 tablespoons chopped onion

1 tablespoon minced jalapeño chile (optional)

Add one can of the drained beans and a little of the broth (about ½ cup) to a food processor and puree. Combine the pureed beans, remaining beans, remaining broth, thyme, bay leaf, and hot pepper sauce in a medium saucepan. Bring to a boil over medium heat. Reduce the heat and simmer 10 minutes for flavors to blend.

Ladle into three bowls and top each serving with one-third of the tomato, onion, and jalapeño chile (if using).

Per serving: Calories 265, Protein 17g, Total fat 3g, Sat fat 0.5g, Trans fat 0g, Cholesterol 2mg, Carbohydrate 40g, Dietary fiber 16g, Sodium 936mg

MIXED SEAFOOD IN
TOMATO BROTH

Makes 3 servings; about 5 cups

When you're sipping this seafood broth, you'll feel like a true gourmet even on your down days.

2 tablespoons minced shallot

1 celery stalk, chopped

½ green or yellow bell pepper, chopped

1 medium red potato, cut into ⅓-inch cubes (about ½ cup)

2 medium Roma tomatoes, chopped (do not seed or peel)

1 bay leaf

¼ teaspoon dried thyme

Generous dash of hot pepper sauce, or to taste

4 cups reduced-sodium chicken broth

½ cup dry white wine

¼ pound medium shrimp, peeled and deveined

¼ pound bay scallops or quartered sea scallops

¼ pound crabmeat, picked through for shells

Chopped fresh flat-leaf parsley, for garnish

Spray a large saucepan with cooking spray. Add the shallot and celery and cook over medium heat, stirring occasionally, until softened, about 3 minutes. Add the bell pepper, potato, tomatoes, bay leaf, thyme, hot pepper sauce, broth, and wine. Bring to a boil. Reduce the heat, cover, and simmer until the vegetables are tender, about 15 minutes.

Add the shrimp and cook until pink, about 3 minutes. Add the scallops and crabmeat and simmer until the scallops are cooked through, about 2 minutes. Discard the bay leaf. Ladle into three bowls and sprinkle with parsley.

Per serving: Calories 231, Protein 27g, Total fat 4g, Sat fat 1g, Trans fat 0g,
Cholesterol 108mg, Carbohydrate 16g, Dietary fiber 2g, Sodium 424mg

ASPARAGUS, CARROT, AND PEAS IN BROTH

Makes 1 serving; about 2 cups

Here's a delicious way to get a variety of the vegetables that provide health-protective phytochemicals.

1 (14-ounce) can reduced-sodium chicken broth

4 asparagus stalks, cut into ½-inch lengths

2 small carrots, cut crosswise into thin slices (about ½ cup)

½ cup frozen green peas

4 fresh mint leaves or 1 teaspoon fresh dill

Bring the broth to a boil in a small saucepan over medium heat. Add the vegetables and return to a boil. Reduce the heat, cover, and simmer until the vegetables are tender, about 10 minutes.

Stack the mint leaves and cut crosswise into thin shreds. Ladle the soup into a bowl and sprinkle with the mint.

Per serving: Calories 148, Protein 10g, Total fat 3g, Sat fat 1g, Trans fat 0g,
Cholesterol 7mg, Carbohydrate 21g, Dietary fiber 6g, Sodium 310mg

EGG DROP SOUP

Makes 2 servings; 2⅓ cups

Egg drop soup from the local Chinese takeout can be extremely high in sodium. Making it yourself is a snap, and avoids that problem.

1 (14-ounce) can reduced-sodium
  chicken broth

2 slices fresh ginger, peeled

4 ounces firm tofu, cubed
  (about ½ cup)

1 cup packed baby spinach leaves or
  shredded napa cabbage

2 egg whites, lightly beaten, or
  ½ cup egg substitute

2 tablespoons minced green onion
  tops or chives

Sriracha sauce (hot chili sauce), to
  taste (see Note)

Salt and freshly ground black
  pepper, to taste

Bring the broth and ginger to a boil in a medium saucepan over medium heat. Add the tofu and spinach and cook until the spinach wilts, about 2 minutes. Reduce the heat so soup just simmers and slowly pour in the egg whites, stirring constantly. Remove from the heat and stir in the green onions. Season with Sriracha sauce, salt, and pepper. Discard the ginger and ladle the soup into two bowls.

Per serving: Calories 91, Protein 11g, Total fat 4g, Sat fat 1g, Trans fat 0g,
Cholesterol 3mg, Carbohydrate 4g, Dietary fiber 0g, Sodium 170mg

Note: *Sriracha (SEE-rah-chah) sauce is the generic name for a very spicy sauce from Thailand that is made of ground hot chiles, vinegar, garlic, sugar, and salt. Use with caution until you determine the amount of heat you prefer. Sriracha sauce is available in Asian markets and with other Asian ingredients in some supermarkets. Refrigerate the sauce after opening.*

ASIAN CHICKEN NOODLE SOUP

Makes 3 servings; about 5½ cups

Using low-carb shirataki tofu noodles changes this chicken soup from the usual high-carb version to one that will spark your taste buds with its different flavor and texture.

4 cups reduced-sodium chicken broth

1 cup chopped zucchini

1 cup chopped red or yellow bell pepper

4 green onions, cut into ½-inch pieces

6 ounces cooked chicken breast, in bite-size pieces

1 (8-ounce) package shirataki tofu noodles, drained, cut into bite-size pieces, prepared according to package directions, and drained again (see page 189)

Salt and freshly ground black pepper, to taste

Hot pepper sauce, to taste

Bring all the ingredients except the noodles and seasonings to a boil over medium heat. Reduce the heat, cover, and simmer until the vegetables are tender, about 10 minutes. Stir in the noodles and bring back to a simmer. Season with salt, black pepper, and hot pepper sauce. Ladle into three bowls and serve.

Per serving: Calories 165, Protein 22g, Total fat 4g, Sat fat 2g, Trans fat 0g, Cholesterol 49mg, Carbohydrate 10g, Dietary fiber 3g, Sodium 195mg

VIETNAMESE SOUP

Makes 2 servings; about 4 cups

The fresh, earthy flavor of cilantro gives this Asian-inspired soup a nice pungency.

3 cups reduced-sodium chicken broth

1 lemongrass stalk, crushed (see Note)

1 cup packed shredded napa cabbage or bok choy leaves

1 small carrot, cut into thin strips

4 ounces cooked chicken breast, shredded (about ⅔ cup)

2 tablespoons shredded fresh basil leaves, preferably Thai basil

2 tablespoons fresh cilantro leaves

2 green onions, cut diagonally into 1-inch pieces

1 tablespoon minced jalapeño or serrano chile, or to taste

Bring the broth and lemongrass to a boil in a medium saucepan over medium heat. Add the cabbage, carrot, and chicken. Boil until the greens are wilted, about 2 minutes. Discard the lemongrass. Ladle into two bowls and top each serving with half the basil, cilantro, and green onions. Add chile to taste.

Per serving: Calories 206, Protein 27g, Total fat 45, Sat fat 2g, Trans fat 0g, Cholesterol 54mg, Carbohydrate 16g, Dietary fiber 5g, Sodium 240mg

Note: *Only the bottom 3 or 4 inches of the lemongrass is used. Crush with a meat mallet. Look for lemongrass with other fresh herbs in the produce section. Lemongrass paste is available in tubes in the produce section of some supermarkets. If lemongrass is not available, a strip of lemon peel can be used for a somewhat similar taste.*

Konjac and Shirataki Tofu Noodles

Konjac, derived from the root of the konjac plant, is a kind of yam that has been eaten in China and Japan for two thousand years. The chemical structure is a very long chain of indigestible, soluble fiber that passes through your GI tract largely unchanged and, therefore, has no calories. It also slows the absorption of sugar, thereby reducing the postmeal insulin response by up to 50 percent.

The root is ground into flour and used to make a variety of noodles and cakes. The noodles have a slight fishy odor that is eliminated when they are mixed with flavorings. Except when made into orzo or pearl pasta, however, they are also quite rubbery, and some people dislike the chewy texture. Konjac is extremely filling, and I like to add it to soup to increase volume and satiety. There are multiple vendors of konjac on the Internet.

Shirataki tofu noodles are made by combining tofu and konjac. Although they have a few more calories than konjac (total of 40 per 8-ounce bag), they are not fishy and are much less chewy. Because they have no flavor, they will take on the taste of whatever they're mixed with and can be used in virtually any soup, with any pasta sauce, or in any casserole. The noodles are packed in water and sold in plastic bags; they need to be kept refrigerated. They are available at some specialty supermarkets or online. For information about where to buy them, go to house-foods.com. Recipes using shirataki tofu noodles can be found on pages 187, 200, 223, and 225.

Judy's Down-Day Salad

Makes 4 to 6 large servings

◇◇◇

This nutrient-dense, antioxidant-enriched, calorie-sparse salad requires a lot of chewing and takes a long time to eat. It will make you think you've really eaten a lot!

1 cup shredded romaine lettuce

1 cup mixed salad greens

1 cup chopped green onions

1 cup sliced mushrooms

1 cup diced green and red pepper

1 cup alfalfa or clover sprouts

1 cup mung-bean sprouts

1 cup sliced carrots

1 cup celery chunks

1 cup shredded baby bok choy

½ cup sliced canned water
    chestnuts

6 fresh asparagus spears, cut in
    ½-inch lengths

3 marinated artichoke hearts,
    drained and sliced

2 hard-cooked egg whites, chopped

Lemon juice or balsamic vinegar, for
    dressing

Wash and dry all the ingredients as necessary. Combine in a large bowl without the dressing and mix well.

Dress with fresh lemon juice (4 calories per tablespoon) or with balsamic vinegar (10 calories per tablespoon) just before serving.

Per serving (without dressing): Calories 93, Protein 7g, Total fat 1g,

Sat fat 0g, Trans fat 0g, Cholesterol 0mg, Carbohydrate 17g,

Dietary fiber 0g, Sodium 120mg

Watermelon and Tomato Salad with Goat Cheese

Makes 1 serving

This combination may sound odd to you, but once you try it you're sure to love it.

2 cups mixed salad greens

1 Roma tomato, quartered

6 (1-inch) watermelon cubes

2 tablespoons low-fat goat cheese, crumbled

2 tablespoons low-fat balsamic vinaigrette dressing, such as Newman's Own

Arrange the greens on a plate. Top with the tomato, watermelon, and goat cheese. Drizzle with the vinaigrette.

Per serving: Calories 126, Protein 5g, Total fat 6g, Sat fat 2g, Trans fat 0g, Cholesterol 7mg, Carbohydrate 14g, Dietary fiber 3g, Sodium 400mg

Variation: *In the winter you can substitute honeydew or cantaloupe for the watermelon.*

salads

GARBANZO BEAN–
SPINACH SALAD

Makes 2 servings

Call them garbanzos or chickpeas, they're still delicious—and oh so good for you.

1 cup cooked or no-salt-added
   canned garbanzo beans, drained
   and rinsed
¼ cup low-fat vinaigrette dressing
   of your choice
1 teaspoon minced garlic

Salt and freshly ground black
   pepper, to taste
3 cups baby spinach leaves
2 Roma tomatoes, cut into wedges
½ small red onion, cut crosswise
   into rings

In a large bowl, toss the beans with the vinaigrette and garlic. Season with salt and pepper. Add half the spinach and toss to combine. Add the remaining spinach and the tomatoes and toss again. Divide the salad between two plates and top with the onion rings.

Per serving: Calories 183, Protein 9g, Total fat 5g, Sat fat 0.4g, Trans fat 0g, Cholesterol 0mg, Carbohydrate 27g, Dietary fiber 8g, Sodium 351mg

WHITE BEAN-ARTICHOKE
HEART SALAD

Makes 2 servings

The marinade from the artichoke hearts makes the dressing for this salad—what could be easier? On your up days, top each salad with 2 tablespoons.

1 (6-ounce) jar marinated artichoke
  hearts

1 (15-ounce) can cannellini or other
  white beans, drained and rinsed

1 large Roma tomato, diced

1 celery stalk, diced

1 tablespoon shredded fresh basil or
  1 teaspoon dried

Freshly ground black pepper, to
  taste

3 cups mixed salad greens

Drain the artichoke hearts and reserve the marinade. Cut the artichoke hearts into quarters and place in a large bowl. Add the beans, tomato, and celery and toss gently to combine. Add the basil and about 1 tablespoon of the marinade. Season with black pepper and toss gently. Let stand at room temperature for 30 minutes for flavors to blend, or cover and refrigerate for up to 8 hours. If refrigerated, bring to room temperature before serving. Divide the greens between two plates, top with the artichoke and bean mixture, and serve.

Per serving: Calories 276, Protein 13g, Total fat 6g, Sat fat 0g, Trans fat 0g, Cholesterol 0mg, Carbohydrate 46g, Dietary fiber 14g, Sodium 807mg

salads

ROMAINE HEARTS WITH
BUTTERMILK DRESSING

Makes 2 servings

The secret to this salad is crisp, chilled lettuce. Halve the lettuce, rinse thoroughly, drain, and refrigerate in a plastic bag for at least one hour before serving.

FOR THE DRESSING:

5 tablespoons reduced-fat
buttermilk

2 tablespoons nonfat mayonnaise

½ teaspoon Dijon mustard

1 garlic clove, minced

1 teaspoon fresh dill or
¼ teaspoon dried

Salt and freshly ground black
pepper, to taste

FOR THE SALAD:

1 head romaine heart, halved
lengthwise

2 Roma tomatoes, diced (do not
seed or peel, but do drain slightly)

¼ cup diced sweet onion

2 tablespoons reduced-fat feta
cheese

Combine all the dressing ingredients in a bowl and whisk until combined. Cover and refrigerate for at least 30 minutes or overnight for the flavors to blend.

Arrange a lettuce half on each of two plates. Drizzle one-fourth of the dressing over each half. Sprinkle with the tomatoes, onion, and cheese and drizzle with more dressing to taste.

Per serving: Calories 73, Protein 5g, Total fat 2g, Sat fat 1g, Trans fat 0g, Cholesterol 4mg, Carbohydrate 12g, Dietary fiber 3g, Sodium 284mg

Broccoli Summer Salad

Makes 3 servings

Blanching the broccoli leaves it crisp-tender but not raw.

1 cup broccoli florets

¼ cup seeded and diced yellow or
orange bell pepper

2 tablespoons chopped red onion

½ cup chopped zucchini

1 cup cherry or grape tomatoes,
halved

2 teaspoons dried basil

1 teaspoon dried oregano

¼ cup store-bought light ranch
dressing of your choice

3 tablespoons crumbled reduced-
fat feta cheese

Salt and freshly ground black
pepper, to taste

Bring a pot of lightly salted water to a boil. Fill a bowl with ice water. Add the broccoli to the boiling water and bring back to a boil. Drain and add the broccoli to the ice water. Drain again and transfer the blanched broccoli to a large serving bowl. Add the bell pepper, onion, zucchini, tomatoes, basil, and oregano. Add the dressing and cheese and toss to combine. Taste and season with salt and pepper, if needed.

Per serving: Calories 112, Protein 4g, Total fat 7g, Sat fat 2g, Trans fat 0g, Cholesterol 15mg, Carbohydrate 8g, Dietary fiber 3g, Sodium 274mg

DICED APPLE AND TUNA SALAD WITH LETTUCE AND CUCUMBER WEDGES

Makes 2 servings

The apple adds a tart crunch to this tasty tuna salad.

2 tablespoons nonfat mayonnaise

1 tablespoon plain nonfat yogurt

1 tablespoon freshly squeezed lime juice

1 small Granny Smith apple, unpeeled, diced

½ cup diced celery

¼ cup minced green onions (green parts only)

1 (6-ounce) can water-packed albacore tuna, drained

6 leaves butter lettuce or red or green leaf lettuce

½ cucumber, peeled and cut into wedges

Combine the mayonnaise, yogurt, and lime juice in a medium bowl. Add the apple, celery, green onions, and tuna. Toss gently until combined.

Line two plates with the lettuce leaves. Divide the salad between the plates and garnish with the cucumber wedges.

Per serving: Calories 165, Protein 23g, Total fat 1g, Sat fat 0g, Trans fat 0g, Cholesterol 26mg, Carbohydrate 17g, Dietary fiber 3g, Sodium 429mg

Edamame and Green Bean Salad

Makes 2 servings

Edamame are fresh soybeans. They are sold either shelled or in their pods. Keep frozen shelled edamame and thin green beans (also called haricots verts) in your freezer for making this salad and also for adding to stir-fries.

1 cup frozen shelled edamame

2 cups thin green beans (haricots verts), fresh or frozen

1 celery stalk, thinly sliced on the diagonal

¼ cup commercial sesame-ginger vinaigrette, such as Newman's Own

2 cups shredded romaine lettuce

Bring a pot of salted water to a boil. Prepare a bowl of ice water. Add the edamame and green beans to the boiling water and boil until the green beans are crisp-tender, 4 to 6 minutes. Drain and add to the ice water to stop the cooking. Then drain thoroughly.

Combine the edamame, green beans, and celery in a medium bowl. Add the dressing and toss to combine. Let marinate at room temperature for 30 minutes, or overnight in the refrigerator. (If refrigerated, bring to room temperature before serving.) Just before serving, add the lettuce and toss the salad to combine.

Per serving: Calories 264, Protein 19g, Total fat 12g, Sat fat 1g, Trans fat 0g, Cholesterol 0mg, Carbohydrate 24g, Dietary fiber 11g, Sodium 277mg

Jicama, Orange, and Arugula Salad

Makes 2 servings

Jicama, also called a Mexican potato or Mexican turnip, is a legume that is eaten raw and crunchy. You can find it in the produce aisle of most supermarkets. Try it in this salad, and I guarantee it will become a staple of your Alternate-Day Diet pantry.

1 large navel orange

1 tablespoon reduced-sodium soy sauce

1 tablespoon balsamic vinegar

1 teaspoon sesame oil

½ small jicama (about 6 ounces), peeled and cut into thin strips

½ sweet onion, cut crosswise and separated into rings

1½ cups lightly packed arugula

Cut the peel and bitter white pith from the orange. Hold the orange over a bowl and separate the segments from the membranes with a thin knife. Squeeze the juice from the membranes into the bowl and add the soy sauce, vinegar, and sesame oil. Whisk to combine.

Combine the orange segments, jicama, and onion in a bowl. Add a little of the dressing and toss gently to combine.

Place the arugula in a second bowl and toss with the remaining dressing. Divide the arugula between two plates and top with the orange, jicama, and onion.

Per serving: Calories 114, Protein 4g, Total fat 1g, Sat fat 0g, Trans fat 0g, Cholesterol 0mg, Carbohydrate 25g, Dietary fiber 8g, Sodium 329mg

SPINACH-COUSCOUS SALAD   *Makes 2 servings*

Couscous is a tiny semolina pasta that is the North African answer to rice. Find it in the same aisle as pasta and rice in your local supermarket.

1½ cups lightly packed baby spinach leaves

1 cup bite-size pieces romaine lettuce

½ English or greenhouse cucumber, unpeeled, sliced

½ small red onion, sliced crosswise into thin rings

½ cup cooked couscous (about ⅓ cup dry), preferably whole-wheat

¼ cup store-bought light ranch dressing

Combine the vegetables and couscous in a large bowl. Toss with the dressing, divide between two plates, and serve.

Per serving: Calories 118, Protein 3g, Total fat 2g, Sat fat 0g, Trans fat 0g, Cholesterol 0mg, Carbohydrate 22g, Dietary fiber 3g, Sodium 391mg

MIXED GREENS TOSSED WITH NOODLES

Makes 2 servings

Using a store-bought low-fat Asian-style dressing makes this salad a quick meal.

1 (8-ounce) package shirataki tofu noodles, drained, cut into bite-size pieces, prepared according to package directions, and drained again (see page 189)

1 (5-ounce) bag salad greens

¼ pound snow peas, blanched until crisp-tender

1 bunch radishes, trimmed and thinly sliced

¼ cup low-fat sesame-ginger vinaigrette, preferably Newman's Own

Rinse the noodles in cold water and drain well. Combine the greens, snow peas, radishes, and noodles in a large bowl. Toss with the salad dressing, divide between two plates, and serve.

Per serving: Calories 100, Protein 5g, Total fat 4g, Sat fat 0.4g, Trans fat 0g, Cholesterol 0mg, Carbohydrate 14g, Dietary fiber 3g, Sodium 292mg

Note: *When combining several cups of salad greens with dressing, it is often easier to toss half the greens and dressing, then add the remaining greens and dressing and toss again.*

CRAB CAKES ON GREENS WITH GREEN BEANS AND TOMATOES

Makes 2 servings

This salad is substantial enough to make a satisfying meal.

FOR THE CRAB CAKES:

8 ounces crabmeat

2 tablespoons nonfat mayonnaise

1 teaspoon Dijon mustard

1 teaspoon freshly squeezed lemon
juice

Pinch of salt

¾ teaspoon Old Bay seasoning
or dash of cayenne

¼ cup soft, fresh whole-wheat
bread crumbs

FOR THE SALAD:

¼ pound thin green beans (haricots
verts), fresh or frozen, steamed
until crisp-tender

2 Roma tomatoes, cut into wedges

4 cups bite-size pieces romaine
lettuce

2 to 3 tablespoons commercial
low-fat Italian vinaigrette

Preheat the oven to 400 degrees. Spray a baking sheet with non-stick cooking spray. Pick over the crabmeat and remove any bits of shell or cartilage. Combine the mayonnaise, mustard, lemon, salt, Old Bay seasoning, and bread crumbs in a medium bowl. Add the crabmeat and mix gently just until combined, being careful not to break up the crabmeat.

Form into 4 rounds. Place on the prepared baking sheet and flatten into patties. Bake on the middle rack of the pre-heated oven for about 15 minutes, until the crab cakes are browned.

While the crab cakes cook, combine the green beans, tomatoes, and lettuce in a large bowl and toss with the dressing. Arrange the salad on two plates and top each serving with two crab cakes.

Per serving: Calories 237, Protein 29g, Total fat 4g, Sat fat 0.4g, Trans fat 0g, Cholesterol 81mg, Carbohydrate 23g, Dietary fiber 5g, Sodium 830mg

Broiled Halibut and Cherry Tomatoes Florentine

Makes 2 servings

The name of this dish may sound exotic but the preparation couldn't be simpler. Serve it as is on your down days and add steamed potatoes garnished with chives for an up-day fish feast.

2 (6-ounce) halibut fillets

6 cherry tomatoes

Salt, freshly ground black pepper,
  and cayenne pepper, to taste

2 garlic cloves, minced

6 to 8 ounces fresh spinach
  (4 cups packed), washed

Salt, to taste

2 lemon wedges

Preheat the broiler. Spray a nonstick baking pan with cooking spray. Arrange the halibut and tomatoes in the pan and season with salt, black pepper, and cayenne. Broil until the halibut is cooked through and no longer translucent in the center, 5 to 10 minutes, depending on the thickness of the fillets.

While the fish cooks, place the garlic in a large saucepan. Add the spinach with the water clinging to its leaves plus 1 tablespoon water. Cook over high heat, stirring occasionally, until the spinach is wilted, about 2 minutes. Season with salt.

Press any water out of the cooked spinach and divide equally between two plates. Arrange the halibut and tomatoes over the spinach. Serve with lemon wedges.

Per serving: Calories 159, Protein 27g, Total fat 3g, Sat fat 0.4g, Trans fat 0g, Cholesterol 36mg, Carbohydrate 6g, Dietary fiber 1g, Sodium 133mg

A Word on Fish and Shellfish

Always try to find the freshest fish possible, either at a fish market or your local supermarket. In most recipes, similar types of fish can be substituted for one another. For example, a mild white fish such as cod could be used in a recipe calling for flounder—another mild white fish. Bring the fresh fish home and refrigerate it as soon as possible. It's best to cook fresh fish the day it is purchased.

If there is not a good source of fresh fish in your area, buy frozen seafood. Make sure the package shows no signs of thawing and refreezing. Look for resealable packages of individually wrapped fillets, which are often available at the large warehouse stores. Frozen fish is convenient to keep on hand, is usually less expensive than fresh, and is often of higher quality.

Many people are afraid of cooking fish. The most common mistake is to overcook it, making the fish dry. The rule is to cook it for about 10 minutes per inch of thickness, measuring at the thickest part. (If the fish is frozen, double the cooking time.) When fish is done, the flesh is no longer translucent (shiny) but opaque or matte in color and should flake when probed with a fork.

Shrimp should be cooked only until it turns pink, 3 to 5 minutes, depending on the size. Fresh shellfish such as clams and mussels are steamed just until the shells open. (Discard any that remain closed.)

SOFT FISH TACOS

Try these tasty, tangy tortillas to add some spice to your down days.

2 (6-ounce) cod or other white fish fillets

4 corn tortillas

½ cup store-bought green or red salsa

2 cups shredded lettuce

¼ cup thinly sliced red onion

½ cup thinly sliced radishes

2 tablespoons fresh cilantro leaves

Bring a shallow pot of lightly salted water to a simmer over medium-low heat. Add the fish and simmer (do not boil) until it is opaque and flakes with a fork, about 10 minutes after the water returns to a simmer. (If the fish is frozen, double the cooking time.) Remove with a spatula and drain.

Heat the tortillas in the microwave for about 30 seconds, until softened. Divide the fish among the tortillas. Top with the salsa, lettuce, onion, radishes, and cilantro.

Per serving: Calories 296, Protein 34g, Total fat 2g, Sat fat 0.4g, Trans fat 0g, Cholesterol 73mg, Carbohydrate 33g, Dietary fiber 5g, Sodium 426mg

Variation: *The fish can also be grilled, steamed, or broiled.*

TROUT WITH CAPERS AND LEMON

Makes 2 servings

◇◇

Lemon and capers are a classic flavor combination.

2 (6-ounce) trout fillets

2 tablespoons capers, rinsed and
   chopped

2 tablespoons freshly squeezed
   lemon juice

Salt and freshly ground black
   pepper, to taste

TO SERVE:

2 cups broccoli florets, steamed
   until crisp-tender

Spray a large nonstick skillet with cooking spray and heat over medium heat. Add the trout and cook until browned on the bottom, about 5 minutes. Carefully turn the trout and add the capers and lemon juice. Season with salt and pepper, cover, and continue cooking until the trout is opaque and flakes with a fork, about 5 minutes. Transfer the trout and broccoli to two plates and serve.

Per serving with broccoli: Calories 260, Protein 38g, Total fat 9g,
Sat fat 3g, Trans fat 0g, Cholesterol 100mg, Carbohydrate 5g,
Dietary fiber 2g, Sodium 334mg

GRILLED FISH WITH PAPAYA-
BELL PEPPER SALSA
Makes 2 servings

As a general rule, fish is cooked for 10 minutes per one inch of thickness, measured at the thickest part. Double the cooking time if the fish is frozen.

FOR THE SALSA:

1 cup papaya cubes

¼ cup diced green or red bell
pepper

2 tablespoons diced red onion

1 garlic clove, minced

2 tablespoons chopped fresh
cilantro

2 tablespoons freshly squeezed
lemon juice

1 teaspoon minced jalapeño chile,
or to taste

Pinch of salt

FOR THE FISH:

2 (about 6-ounce) cod, snapper, or
flounder fillets

Salt and freshly ground black
pepper, to taste

Combine all the salsa ingredients in a medium bowl. (Salsa can be prepared up to a day ahead and refrigerated. Allow it to come to room temperature before serving.)

Preheat a grill or broiler. Spray the fish and the grill rack with cooking spray. Season the fish with salt and pepper and grill about 10 minutes, until it is opaque and flakes with a fork.

Transfer the fish to two plates and top with the salsa.

Per serving: Calories 182, Protein 31g, Total fat 1g, Sat fat 0.3g, Trans fat 0g, Cholesterol 73mg, Carbohydrate 11g, Dietary fiber 2g, Sodium 97mg

ROASTED SALMON, ASPARAGUS, BELL PEPPER, AND MUSHROOMS

Makes 2 servings

Wild salmon is not only delicious but also filled with omega-3 fatty acids, which your body can't make for itself.

6 asparagus spears, ends trimmed

1 yellow or orange bell pepper, seeded and cut lengthwise into 8 pieces

6 medium cremini (brown) mushrooms, stems removed

Salt and freshly ground black pepper, to taste

¼ teaspoon dried thyme

2 (4-ounce) salmon fillets, preferably wild

2 lime wedges, for serving

Preheat the oven to 450 degrees. Arrange the asparagus, bell pepper, and mushrooms in a 13 × 9-inch nonstick baking pan. Spray with cooking spray and season with salt and pepper. Sprinkle with thyme. Cover with foil and roast for 10 minutes. Uncover and roast 10 minutes longer, or until the vegetables are crisp-tender.

While the vegetables cook, spray an 8-inch-square nonstick baking pan with cooking spray. Arrange the salmon fillets in the pan, season with salt and pepper, and roast for about 10 minutes, until the salmon is no longer translucent in the center.

Arrange one piece of salmon and half the vegetables on each of two plates. Serve with lime wedges.

Per serving: Calories 248, Protein 26g, Total fat 12g, Sat fat 3g, Trans fat 0g, Cholesterol 75mg, Carbohydrate 9g, Dietary fiber 3g, Sodium 58mg

VEGETABLE-TOPPED FISH IN THE MICROWAVE, MEXICAN-STYLE

Makes 1 serving

An easy moist fish dish with a lot of flavor, this is perfect for summer because it cooks quickly and you don't have to turn on the oven.

1 (about 6-ounce) cod, snapper, or flounder fillet

2 tablespoons nonfat or reduced-fat mayonnaise

1 teaspoon freshly squeezed lime juice

1 green onion, finely chopped

½ Roma tomato, diced

2 tablespoons minced red bell pepper

1 teaspoon minced jalapeño chile, or to taste

Spray a small microwave-safe dish with cooking spray. Place the fillet in the dish and set aside. Combine the remaining ingredients in a small bowl. Spread over the fish. Cover dish with plastic wrap, venting one corner. Microwave on high power for 2 minutes. Check the fish with a fork to see if it flakes and is opaque. If not, re-cover and microwave for 30 seconds more, then check again. Transfer to a plate and serve.

Per serving: Calories 176, Protein 31g, Total fat 1g, Sat fat 0g, Trans fat 0g Cholesterol 73mg, Carbohydrate 10g, Dietary fiber 1g, Sodium 307mg

Seared Scallops in Tarragon Sauce

Makes 2 servings

When you taste this creamy sauce you'll never believe it could be so low in calories. For a filling up-day dinner, spoon the scallops and sauce over whole-wheat noodles.

For the Sauce:

½ cup reduced-fat chicken broth

1 ½ teaspoons cornstarch

2 tablespoons nonfat cream
  cheese

1 tablespoon minced fresh tarragon
  or 1 teaspoon dried

2 tablespoons minced fresh chives

Salt, to taste

For the Scallops:

2 teaspoons canola oil

¾ pound sea scallops, patted dry

1 tablespoon freshly squeezed lime
  juice

To Serve:

2 cups fresh young green beans,
  steamed until crisp-tender

Make the sauce: Whisk a little of the broth and the cornstarch together in a small saucepan. Whisk in the remaining broth, add the cream cheese, and cook over medium heat, stirring, until the cheese has melted and the sauce is thickened and bubbly. Stir in the tarragon and chives, season with salt, and remove from the heat.

To cook the scallops, heat the oil in a medium nonstick skillet over high heat. Add the scallops and sauté carefully, so they don't break, until golden, about 2 minutes. Stir in the lime juice. Add the scallops to the sauce and divide between two plates. Serve with the green beans on the side.

Per serving with green beans: Calories 225, Protein 32g, Total fat 6g, Sat fat 1g, Trans fat 0g, Cholesterol 60mg, Carbohydrate 8g, Dietary fiber 0g, Sodium 411mg

CHICKEN WITH ARTICHOKE HEARTS ITALIANO
Makes 4 servings

Who said you can't eat Italian on a diet? This tasty chicken dish will give you a big lift on your down days.

1/2 cup chopped onion

1/4 cup water

2 garlic cloves, minced

1 pound boneless, skinless chicken
  breasts, cut into thin strips

4 ounces cremini (brown)
  mushrooms, sliced (about
  3/4 cup)

1 (14-ounce) can artichoke hearts,
  drained, rinsed, and quartered

1 (14.5-ounce) can diced tomatoes
  with juice

1 teaspoon dried oregano

2 teaspoons dried basil

Freshly ground black pepper, to
  taste

Combine the onion and water in a large nonstick skillet over medium heat. Cook, stirring occasionally, until the water evaporates. Add the garlic and chicken and cook, stirring occasionally, until the chicken is browned, about 5 minutes. Add the mushrooms, artichoke hearts, tomatoes with juice, oregano, and basil. Season with black pepper.

Stir to combine the ingredients, cover, and simmer until the chicken and vegetables are tender, about 10 minutes. Divide among four plates and serve.

Per serving: Calories 217, Protein 32g, Total fat 2g, Sat fat 0.4g, Trans fat 0g, Cholesterol 66mg, Carbohydrate 19g, Dietary fiber 6g, Sodium 804mg

SHREDDED CHICKEN AND VEGETABLES IN LETTUCE LEAF CUPS *Makes 2 servings*

Here's a typical Chinese restaurant dish adapted for down-day dieting.

6 ounces cooked chicken breast, shredded

1 tablespoon hoisin sauce

1 tablespoon reduced-sodium soy sauce

Sriracha sauce (hot chili sauce), to taste (see Note page 186)

2 cups (8 ounces) bean sprouts

2 celery stalks, cut into thin diagonal slices

10 snow peas (about 2 ounces) each cut into 3 diagonal pieces

6 to 8 large lettuce leaves, such as romaine or red or green leaf lettuce

2 green onions, minced, for garnish

Combine the chicken, hoisin sauce, soy sauce, and Sriracha sauce in a medium bowl.

Bring a small pot of water to a boil.

Place the bean sprouts in a strainer; set in the sink or over a large bowl.

Add the celery and snow peas to the boiling water and return to a boil. Immediately pour over the bean sprouts in the strainer. Drain well and add to the chicken. Mix well.

Fill the lettuce leaf cups with the chicken mixture and garnish with the green onions.

Per serving: Calories 174, Protein 25g, Total fat 2g, Sat fat 0.4g, Trans fat 0g, Cholesterol 50mg, Carbohydrate 16g, Dietary fiber 4g, Sodium 498mg

CHICKEN WITH PINEAPPLE, BELL PEPPERS, AND ONIONS

Makes 2 servings

Think of this as a sweet-and-sour stir-fry made without a wok.

6 ounces boneless, skinless chicken breast, cut into ½-inch pieces

1 large carrot, cut on the diagonal into thin slices

About ¼ cup reduced-sodium chicken broth

1 (8-ounce) can unsweetened pineapple chunks in juice, drained, juice reserved

1 large green bell pepper, seeded and cut into thin strips

4 green onions, cut into 1-inch lengths

1 tablespoon cider vinegar

1 tablespoon grated fresh ginger

½ tablespoon cornstarch mixed with 2 tablespoons water

Salt and freshly ground black pepper, to taste

Spray a nonstick skillet with a lid with cooking spray and heat over medium heat. Add the chicken and cook, stirring and turning occasionally, until browned, about 5 minutes. Add the carrot and cook about 3 minutes. Stir in the broth, reserved pineapple juice, and bell pepper. Cover and simmer until the chicken and vegetables are tender, about 5 minutes.

Stir in the pineapple, green onions, vinegar, and ginger. Stir in the cornstarch mixture and cook, stirring, until bubbly and thickened, about 2 minutes. Season with salt and black pepper and serve at once.

Per serving: Calories 236, Protein 23g, Total fat 2g, Sat fat 0.5g, Trans fat 0g, Cholesterol 50mg, Carbohydrate 34g, Dietary fiber 5g, Sodium 114mg

SESAME-CRUSTED BAKED CHICKEN BREASTS ON NAPA CABBAGE

Makes 2 servings

This is a tasty, Asian-inspired variation on oven-baked "fried" chicken.

FOR THE CHICKEN:

1 tablespoon reduced-sodium soy sauce

1 egg white, lightly beaten

1 teaspoon five-spice powder

1 garlic clove, minced

2 (3- to 4-ounce) boneless, skinless chicken breast halves

2 tablespoons white sesame seeds

FOR THE CABBAGE:

½ small head napa cabbage, shredded (3 cups)

1 tablespoon water or reduced-sodium chicken broth

1 tablespoon reduced-sodium soy sauce

1 tablespoon unseasoned rice wine vinegar, or to taste

To make the chicken, combine the soy sauce, egg white, five-spice powder, and garlic in a shallow bowl. Add the chicken and turn to coat. Let stand while the oven preheats to 425 degrees.

Spray a small nonstick baking pan with cooking spray. Spread the sesame seeds in another shallow bowl. Dip the meaty side of the chicken in the sesame seeds to coat. Arrange the chicken in the baking pan, seeded side up. Bake for about 25 minutes, until the chicken is cooked through and the juices run clear.

While the chicken is baking, spray a large skillet or wok with cooking spray and heat over high heat. Add the cabbage and water and cook, covered, tossing occasionally, until the cabbage is crisp-tender, about 3 minutes. Season with soy sauce and vinegar.

Divide the cabbage between two plates and top each serving with a chicken breast.

Per serving: Calories 289, Protein 45g, Total fat 6g, Sat fat 1g, Trans fat 0g, Cholesterol 99mg, Carbohydrate 12g, Dietary fiber 5g, Sodium 630mg

ROASTED TURKEY MEATBALLS IN CREAMY YOGURT SAUCE   *Makes 4 servings*

◇◇

The yogurt sauce gives these low-fat meatballs a Middle Eastern tang. For an up-day treat, serve the meatballs and sauce on a bed of whole-wheat couscous.

FOR THE MEATBALLS:

1 pound extra-lean ground turkey

2 tablespoons minced onion

1 garlic clove, minced

1 egg white or 2 tablespoons egg
   substitute

½ teaspoon salt

1 teaspoon dried thyme

Dash of cayenne pepper

FOR THE SAUCE:

1 cup reduced-sodium chicken broth

1 tablespoon cornstarch

¼ cup plain nonfat yogurt

1 tablespoon chopped fresh mint

1 teaspoon chopped fresh oregano

1 tablespoon freshly grated lemon
   zest

Salt and freshly ground black
   pepper, to taste

TO SERVE:

4 cups fresh sugar snap peas,
   steamed until crisp-tender

To make the meatballs, preheat the oven to 500 degrees. Spray a large nonstick rimmed baking sheet with cooking spray. Combine the turkey, onion, garlic, egg white, salt, thyme, and cayenne in a medium bowl. Form the mixture into small balls, using about 1 tablespoon for each. Arrange on the prepared pan and bake for about 10 minutes, until lightly browned.

While the meatballs are cooking, make the sauce: Whisk a little of the broth together with the cornstarch in a small saucepan and stir until smooth. Whisk in the remaining broth. Cook over medium heat, stirring, until bubbly and thickened, 2 to 3 minutes. Stir in remaining ingredients and remove from the heat.

Transfer the meatballs to a serving dish, top with the yogurt sauce, and serve with the sugar snap peas as a side dish.

Per serving: Calories 231, Protein 33g, Total fat 3g, Sat fat 0.5g, Trans fat 0g, Cholesterol 56mg, Carbohydrate 20g, Dietary fiber 5g, Sodium 433mg

TURKEY CUTLETS WITH THYME-MUSTARD SAUCE
Makes 2 servings

The tryptophan in the turkey will give you that same satisfied feeling you have after Thanksgiving dinner.

2 (3- to 4-ounce) turkey cutlets

1/2 teaspoon dried thyme

Salt and freshly ground black pepper, to taste

About 3/4 cup reduced-sodium chicken broth

2 baby bok choy, halved lengthwise

1 teaspoon Dijon mustard

1/2 teaspoon cornstarch

Place the turkey between 2 sheets of plastic wrap and pound the cutlets with a meat mallet until about 1/8 inch thick. Season with the thyme, salt, and pepper.

Spray a large nonstick skillet with cooking spray and heat over medium heat. Add the turkey and cook until browned on the bottom, about 2 minutes. Turn and add 1/2 cup of the broth and the bok choy. Reduce the heat, cover, and simmer until the bok choy is crisp-tender, about 3 minutes.

Transfer a turkey cutlet and 2 bok choy halves to each of two plates and keep warm. Whisk together the mustard, cornstarch, and 2 tablespoons of the remaining broth in a small bowl and add to the liquid in the skillet. Cook, stirring, until bubbly and thickened, 2 to 3 minutes, adding more broth if needed. Spoon the sauce over the cutlets and serve.

Per serving: Calories 166, Protein 27g, Total fat 3g, Sat fat 1g, Trans fat 0g, Cholesterol 51mg, Carbohydrate 11g, Dietary fiber 4g, Sodium 432mg

TURKEY-STUFFED BELL PEPPERS WITH AN ITALIAN ACCENT *Makes 2 servings*

You'll be surprised how filling these stuffed peppers are.

2 medium red, green, or other color bell peppers, tops removed, seeded and cored

6 ounces extra-lean ground turkey

1/2 cup chopped onion

1/2 cup chopped celery

1 garlic clove, minced

4 ounces fresh mushrooms, chopped (about 1 cup)

1/2 cup frozen green peas, thawed

1 1/2 teaspoons fennel seed

2 tablespoons chopped fresh basil or 1 tablespoon dried

1 teaspoon chopped fresh oregano or 1/2 teaspoon dried

1 tablespoon cider vinegar

1/2 cup prepared tomato sauce

1/4 cup water

2 tablespoons freshly grated Parmesan cheese

Preheat the oven to 375 degrees. Spray a small baking dish just large enough to hold the bell peppers with cooking spray.

Bring a pot of lightly salted water to a boil. Drop the bell peppers into the boiling water and cook for 5 minutes. Drain and rinse in cold water.

Combine the turkey, onion, celery, and garlic in a large skillet and cook over medium heat, stirring to break up the meat, until the turkey is browned. Add the mushrooms and cook until softened, about 5 minutes. Stir in the peas, fennel seed, basil, oregano, and vinegar.

Stuff the bell peppers with the turkey mixture. Place in the prepared dish and pour the tomato sauce and water around the peppers. Cover with foil and bake for about 30 minutes, until the peppers are tender. Uncover, sprinkle with the cheese, and bake for another 5 minutes. Transfer the bell peppers to plates and spoon the cooking liquid over them.

Per serving: Calories 220, Protein 23g, Total fat 3g, Sat fat 1g, Trans fat 0g, Cholesterol 35mg, Carbohydrate 24g, Dietary fiber 6g, Sodium 219mg

TURKEY AND WHITE BEAN CHILI

Makes 3 servings

Making chili with turkey and white beans gives it a new twist. The great thing about spices is that they add a lot of flavor without any calories.

6 ounces extra-lean ground turkey

½ cup chopped onion

1 garlic clove, minced

½ cup seeded and chopped green bell pepper

1 tablespoon minced serrano chile, or to taste

1 (14.5-ounce) can no-salt-added diced tomatoes with juice

1 (15-ounce) can white beans such as cannellini, navy, or great northern, drained and rinsed

1 cup water

1 tablespoon chili powder

1 teaspoon ground cumin

½ teaspoon dried oregano

½ teaspoon dried basil

Combine the turkey, onion, and garlic in a large saucepan and cook over medium heat, stirring to break up the meat, until the turkey is browned. Add the bell pepper, chile, tomatoes with their juice, beans, water, chili powder, cumin, oregano, and basil. Reduce the heat, cover, and simmer until the onion is tender, about 20 minutes.

Per serving: Calories 210, Protein 23g, Total fat 2g, Sat fat 0g, Trans fat 0g, Cholesterol 27mg, Carbohydrate 34g, Dietary fiber 11g, Sodium 589mg

Variation: *For a different texture, substitute 6 ounces of cubed turkey or chicken breast for the ground turkey.*

GRILLED PORK TENDERLOIN, ONION, AND BELL PEPPERS

Makes 4 servings

Pork tenderloin is very lean and works even for a down-day dinner.

1 (about 1-pound) pork tenderloin

Salt and freshly ground black
pepper, to taste

2 large bell peppers, preferably
different colors, seeded and cut
lengthwise into eighths

1 large Vidalia or other sweet onion,
cut crosswise into thick slices and
separated into rings

2 teaspoons chopped fresh oregano
or thyme or 1 teaspoon dried

4 lime wedges, to serve

Preheat a grill. Remove the silverskin (thick connective tissue) and any fat from the pork with a sharp, pointed knife. Spray the pork and grill rack with cooking spray. Season the pork with salt and pepper and grill over medium-high heat for 20 to 25 minutes, turning two or three times. When done the internal temperature should read 160 degrees on an instant-read thermometer. Cover with foil and let stand for 10 minutes to let it cool slightly.

While the pork is standing, spray a grill basket with cooking spray. Add the bell peppers and onion and grill, stirring occasionally, until the vegetables are slightly charred and crisp-tender, 5 to 10 minutes. Cut the pork into long thin strips and toss with the bell pepper mixture and oregano, adding salt and black pepper as needed.

Divide among four plates and serve with lime wedges.

Per serving: Calories 173, Protein 25g, Total fat 4g, Sat fat 1g, Trans fat 0g,
Cholesterol 74mg, Carbohydrate 9g, Dietary fiber 2g, Sodium 60mg

main dishes

Variations: *Yucatán Pork Tenderloin: Rub the pork with 1 table-spoon annatto paste mixed with 1 tablespoon lime juice. Southwest-ern Pork Tenderloin: Rub the pork with 1 to 2 tablespoons of a dry Southwestern rub, preferably one without salt.*

VEGETABLE-STUFFED PORTOBELLO MUSHROOMS
Makes 2 servings

These giant mushrooms are so meaty that you may think you're eating a steak!

2 large portobello mushrooms

¼ cup diced onion

¾ cup seeded and finely chopped green bell pepper

1 small Asian eggplant, with skin, diced

½ cup reduced-sodium chicken broth or as needed

1 Roma tomato, diced (do not seed or peel)

¼ teaspoon ground cumin

¼ teaspoon ground cinnamon

¼ teaspoon sweet smoky Spanish paprika or ⅛ teaspoon ground chipotle chile

Salt and freshly ground black pepper, to taste

Preheat the oven to 400 degrees. Spray a nonstick baking pan just large enough to hold the mushrooms with cooking spray. Remove the stems from the mushrooms and dice the stems. Scrape off the gills with a spoon and discard the gills. Arrange the mushrooms in a single layer in the prepared pan and bake, stem side down, for 10 minutes.

While the mushrooms bake, spray a medium nonstick skillet

with cooking spray and heat over medium heat. Add the onion, bell pepper, diced mushroom stems, and eggplant and cook until softened, moistening with the broth as needed. Stir in the tomato, cumin, cinnamon, and paprika. Season with salt and pepper and cook until the liquid is absorbed.

Turn the mushrooms stem side up and fill with the vegetable mixture. Return to the oven and bake 10 more minutes, until browned.

Per serving: Calories 136, Protein 9g, Total fat 1g, Sat fat 0.3g, Trans fat 0g, Cholesterol 1mg, Carbohydrate 25g, Dietary fiber 10g, Sodium 83mg

VEGETABLE STIR-FRY   *Makes 2 servings*

The variety of vegetables combined with the noodles in this stir-fry provide a variety of tastes and textures that will keep your taste buds satisfied on your down days.

4 green onions, cut diagonally into 1-inch lengths

1 garlic clove, minced

1/4 pound small green beans or snow peas

1/4 small head napa cabbage, shredded (about 3/4 cup)

1 bok choy, cut crosswise into thin slices

2 to 3 tablespoons reduced-sodium chicken broth

3/4 pound bean sprouts

1 teaspoon cornstarch mixed with 2 tablespoons reduced-sodium soy sauce

Sriracha sauce (hot chili sauce), to taste (see Note page 186)

1 (8-ounce) package shirataki tofu noodles, drained, cut into bite-size pieces, prepared according to package directions and drained again (see page 189)

Spray a wok or large skillet with cooking spray and heat over high heat. Add the green onions and stir-fry about 1 minute. Add the garlic and green beans and stir-fry about 2 minutes. Add the cabbage and bok choy and about 2 tablespoons of the broth. Cover and steam until the vegetables are crisp-tender, about 1 minute. Add the bean sprouts and toss to combine. Add the cornstarch mixture and Sriracha sauce. Cook, stirring, until the sauce is bubbly and thickened, 2 to 3 minutes. Stir in the noodles and heat through. Divide between two plates and serve.

Per serving: Calories 177, Protein 15g, Total fat 2g, Sat fat 0g, Trans fat 0g, Cholesterol 0mg, Carbohydrate 33g, Dietary fiber 15g, Sodium 325mg

Variations: *About ½ cup shredded cooked chicken or diced tofu can be added with the noodles, adding about 100 calories.*

ZUCCHINI RIBBONS WITH NO-COOK TOMATO SAUCE

Makes 1 serving

The recipe can be doubled. Adding one tablespoon freshly grated Parmesan cheese will add only 23 calories.

3 medium Roma tomatoes (about 10 ounces), diced

¼ cup shredded fresh basil

1 tablespoon minced garlic

2 teaspoons cider vinegar, or to taste

Pinch of hot pepper flakes

Salt and freshly ground black pepper, to taste

2 (6- to 8-ounce) zucchini

1 tablespoon freshly grated Parmesan or reduced-fat feta cheese (optional)

Combine the tomatoes, basil, garlic, vinegar, hot pepper flakes, salt, and black pepper in a large bowl.

Trim the ends off the zucchini. Cut a thin slice of peel from two opposite sides of each zucchini. Using a sharp knife or a mandoline, cut each zucchini lengthwise into thin slices. Don't worry if some slices break or are slightly uneven. Stack the slices into piles and cut lengthwise down the middle. Bring 2 to 3 inches of water to a boil in a pot with a steamer basket (the water should not touch the bottom of the basket). Spread the zucchini in the basket and cover the pot. Steam for about 3 minutes, until the zucchini is just crisp-tender. Immediately toss the zucchini with the sauce and serve. Sprinkle the cheese on top if desired.

Per serving: Calories 116, Protein 7g, Total fat 1g, Sat fat 0g, Trans fat 0g, Cholesterol 0mg, Carbohydrate 25g, Dietary fiber 8g, Sodium 36mg

Variations: *When flavorful fresh tomatoes are unavailable, substitute 1 (14.5-ounce) can drained diced tomatoes or use a commercial pasta sauce.*

PASTA CARBONARA WITH SHIRATAKI TOFU NOODLES
Makes 2 servings

1 (8-ounce) package shirataki tofu noodles (see page 189)

1 tablespoon minced green onion

1 tablespoon real bacon bits, finely minced

2 tablespoons freshly grated Parmesan cheese

1 tablespoon cheese-flavored Molly McButter (optional)

1 egg, lightly beaten in a bowl large enough to hold the noodles

1 tablespoon minced fresh flat-leaf parsley

Place the noodles in a colander and rinse them under cold water. Boil in 1 quart of water for 3 minutes to remove any fishy odor. Return to the colander and drain. Squeeze out any excess water by pressing on the noodles in the colander with a paper towel. Cut the noodles into 3- to 4-inch lengths with kitchen scissors.

Coat a large frying pan with non-stick cooking spray. Over high heat, stir in the green onion and bacon bits and sauté about 1 minute, until the green onion is softened. Add the noodles and cook, stirring constantly, until heated through. Add the Parmesan cheese and Molly McButter, if using, and continue stirring until the noodles are steaming hot.

Remove from the heat and transfer to the bowl with the egg. With a fork, stir to mix thoroughly and cook the egg. Stir in the parsley and serve at once.

Per serving: Calories 94, Protein 8g, Total fat 5g, Sat fat 2g, Trans fat 0g, Cholesterol 1mg, Carbohydrate 4g, Dietary fiber 2g, Sodium 253mg

Chinese Vegetables with Shirataki Tofu Noodles

Makes 2 large servings

2 cups reduced-sodium chicken broth

2 garlic cloves, minced

1 tablespoon grated fresh ginger

1 tablespoon cornstarch

2 stalks celery, thinly sliced on the diagonal

1 bok choy, thinly sliced crosswise

2 cups fresh snow pea pods

½ cup thinly sliced carrots

1 (8-ounce) can sliced bamboo shoots, drained and rinsed, or

1 (8-ounce) can sliced water chestnuts, drained and rinsed

2 cups fresh bean sprouts

1 (8-ounce) package shirataki noodles, cooked according to package directions (optional)

Salt, pepper, and soy sauce, to taste

Put the chicken broth, garlic, ginger, and cornstarch in a blender and blend on high speed for 10 seconds. Transfer the mixture to a 12-inch deep-sided frying pan and bring to a boil over medium heat. Add the celery, bok choy, snow pea pods, carrots, bamboo shoots, and bean sprouts and bring back to a gentle boil, cook for 3 to 5 minutes, or until crisp-tender or to your liking. Stir in the cooked noodles and heat through but do not overcook. Season with salt, pepper, and soy sauce and serve immediately.

Per serving (without noodles): Calories 213, Protein 17g, Total fat 3g, Sat fat 1g, Trans fat 0g, Cholesterol 4mg, Carbohydrate 38g, Dietary fiber 13g, Sodium 452mg

(with noodles): Calories 233, Protein 18g, Total fat 3.5g, Sat fat 1g, Trans fat 0g, Cholesterol 7mg, Carbohydrate 38g, Dietary fiber 15g, Sodium 467mg

Don's Stir-Fry

Makes 2 servings

Use other low-cal vegetables of your choice, and vary the flavorings with herbs and spices. If you like curry, add a tablespoon of curry powder to the stir-fry when you return the vegetables to the pan.

2 cups broccoli florets

2 onions, sliced

2 cups cut-up asparagus spears

1 cup low-sodium chicken broth

2 garlic cloves

1 tablespoon peeled and sliced fresh
  ginger

1 tablespoon cornstarch

Spray a wok or a large sauté pan with nonstick spray. When the pan is hot, add the broccoli, onions, and asparagus, and stir-fry until they soften and begin to brown. Remove the vegetables from the pan.

Combine the chicken broth, garlic, and ginger in the container of a blender and pulse until the garlic and ginger are chopped fine. Add the cornstarch and stir well.

Pour the chicken broth mixture into the hot pan, bring to a boil, and boil, stirring, just until the cornstarch thickens the liquid. Return the vegetables to the pan and reheat in the broth mixture. Serve at once.

Per serving: Calories 148, Protein 9g, Total fat 1g, Sat fat 0.5g, Trans fat 0g,
Cholesterol 2mg, Carbohydrate 30g, Dietary fiber 8g, Sodium 82mg

12.

Frequently Asked Questions

Q. *When did you first describe the pattern of eating 20 percent/100 percent on alternate days?*

A. I filed a patent application on August 12, 2003, called a "priority date," and a formal application on May 14, 2004, titled "Process for Weight Control and Longevity Extension Through Dietary Management." My colleagues and I conducted our Asthma Study, which was the first time using a version of the Alternate-Day Diet on humans, in 2004. The results were published in 2006.

Q. *Is this a fasting diet?*

A. No. It is not. It is about eating significantly less than normal on alternate days, but it is not a fast, although it is certainly possible to eat 0 calories on the restrictive days. The term my patients and I initially came up with to describe the pattern was "up day, down day." And many online blogs still refer to it as the

Johnson Up-Day, Down-Day Diet or simply the Up-Day, Down-Day Diet.

Q. I've heard that there are people who don't approve of this diet. What are their objections?

A. Generally speaking, the people who don't like the Alternate-Day Diet fall into one of the following categories:

1. People who believe you should not drastically lower calorie intake—a notion with which we agree, if you are doing this on a *daily* basis, because there is too much loss of lean body mass (muscle) with very low-calorie diets.
2. People who have had anorexia or bulimia and have been taught in therapy that "starving and bingeing" behavior is bad for you. We certainly agree that anyone with an eating disorder should seek professional counseling before starting any new diet, but we disagree with the characterization of the Alternate-Day Diet as starving and bingeing. We advise people to eat to the point of satisfaction (but not beyond) on the up day and to adjust their down-day intake to a level they can tolerate to ensure long-term maintenance of the pattern. Our broad experience is that this pattern creates a gradual increase in control over intake, not the aggravation of eating disorders.
3. People who cannot tolerate the feeling of mild hunger, even intermittently. These people, of course, are usually unsuccessful on any diet.
4. People who claim not to be able to limit themselves to a shake or other simple food even on alternate days. Again, these people are usually unsuccessful on any diet.

5. People who don't understand or accept the science behind the Alternate-Day Diet even though abundant evidence confirms the health benefits of calorie restriction, as well as the maintenance of metabolic rate and of muscle mass with the alternate-day pattern.
6. People with a bias in favor of other types of diets, such as "low carb." Despite the evidence that all diets eventually fail, some people believe that since they have lost weight on Atkins, that's all they need. However, the science of nutrition has shown the importance of a mainly plant-based source of calories.

Q. *What is the biggest difference you've seen between the time when you created what was originally known as the Johnson Up-Day, Down-Day Diet (aka the Alternate-Day Diet) and today?*

A. The degree of acceptance. People throughout the world are now using this diet in one form or another. In the beginning, there was a great deal of skepticism on the part of the public as well as some scientists. However, since the publication of the results of our Asthma Study in 2006, there have been many other papers that confirm our results.

Q. *What new information has been discovered recently about the benefits of an alternate-day calorie-restriction diet?*

A. Recent studies confirm our earlier findings that you lose much less muscle on the Alternate-Day Diet than when you cut your calories every day. This means that when you lose weight on the Alternate-Day Diet, your physical strength is maintained. You also look better and your muscles are more defined.

One study suggested that eating foods with a higher fat level on your down days may help to reduce hunger. And other findings indicate the Alternate-Day Diet improves factors that are risks for heart disease, such as high blood pressure and cholesterol.

Q. Is it true that the SIRT1 gene, which you refer to as the "skinny gene," is the primary cause of the health benefits described in the book?

A. There has been some debate about what specific genes are turned on when calories are restricted, but it is now certain that activating SIRT1 is the initiating event. It turns on genes that reduce fat storage and has several other effects that lead to the benefits of disease prevention (including cancer, heart disease, and diabetes), and a healthier metabolism.

Q. I think I have low blood sugar. Is the Alternate-Day Diet safe for me?

A. Hypoglycemia, or low blood sugar, occurs in two forms: reactive and fasting. Reactive hypoglycemia means that two to four hours after eating high-carbohydrate foods, the blood sugar drops too low, producing shakiness, anxiety, sweating, extreme hunger, and palpitations. This is the result of excess insulin release, which drives the blood sugar down. The treatment is to avoid high-glycemic carbohydrates (white flour, rice, potatoes) and sugar by eating low-glycemic foods (vegetables and whole grains) as well as protein- and fat-containing foods, and to eat every three hours. Fasting hypoglycemia is often associated with certain medications, excess alcohol, and with some critical illnesses, and is diagnosed with blood sugar testing after a period of fasting.

If you believe you might be hypoglycemic, you should consult your physician. While symptoms of reactive hypoglycemia can be severe, some people who feel they are experiencing hypoglycemia may not actually have low blood sugar and instead might be experiencing symptoms of "feeling bad," such as lightheadedness or mental sluggishness. In practice, no one on the Alternate-Day Diet has complained of low blood sugar on the down day when they were using a shake. If you have been diagnosed with hypoglycemia or believe you have hypoglycemia, you should discuss the diet with your physician. You may also wish to buy a glucometer and test your own blood sugar. The OneTouch Ultra Mini costs less than $20, and learning to use it can give you a much better idea of how your blood sugar is responding to what you eat or don't eat.

Q. *I have hypoglycemia. I feel faint and dizzy when I don't eat because my blood sugar drops, so I can't do this diet. What should I do?*

A. The symptoms of weakness, faintness, and dizziness are rarely caused by hypoglycemia. They are usually due to dehydration and can be alleviated by drinking more fluids.

Q. *I am diabetic. Can I follow the Alternate-Day Diet?*

A. If you are Type 1 diabetic, it would be too difficult to maintain glycemic control without hypoglycemic episodes and I would advise you not to do the diet.

Type 2 diabetics vary across a broad range in their degree of insulin resistance. Some, especially those controlled by diet, should have no problem. If you are a Type 2 diabetic (90 percent of all diabetics) and are using drugs such as metformin (Glucophage) or rosiglitazone (Avandia) that act by reducing insulin resistance, you should have no low blood sugar problem on the down day. The Alternate-Day Diet reduces insulin resistance, especially if you lose weight, so over time, your medication requirement may be reduced. Before you start this or any diet, however, you should consult the doctor who manages your diabetes.

If you are taking medications that lower blood sugar by increasing insulin release or insulin itself, you would have difficulty controlling your blood sugar, and I would advise you not to do this diet.

Q. *Has any other disease been treated with the Alternate-Day Diet?*

A. Our Asthma Study showed marked improvement in airway function, and unheard-of reduction (up to 90 percent) in oxidative stress markers, which are the free radicals that cause disease.

Q. *Will the diet affect my medications?*

A. First, *everyone* should consult a doctor before starting any diet. In general, however, the Alternate-Day Diet will not affect your medications. If you are using a medication to lower blood sugar (as for diabetes), you will need to closely monitor your blood sugar.

Q. *Does this diet have any side effects?*

A. I have had no reports of it. My main concern would be experiencing dehydration on the down day because of inadequate fluid intake. Many people are mildly or moderately under-hydrated in normal circumstances, so it is critical to take in the equivalent of 2.5 liters of calorie-free liquids per day. You may not actually feel thirsty when you are exerting yourself and losing water rapidly. And older people may not have a sufficient sense of thirst to avoid dehydration. For these reasons it is important to preempt dehydration by intentionally drinking calorie-free liquids throughout the day. Extreme dehydration occurs mainly in children and old people during very hot weather, but minor dehydration can make you feel tired, weak, and irritable. If your urine is clear or very pale yellow, you are adequately hydrated.

Q. *Does the Alternate-Day Diet cause loss of muscle?*

A. The loss of any significant amount of weight inevitably causes some loss of lean body mass (muscle). However, I believe that the Alternate-Day Diet preserves lean body mass more than daily weight-loss diets because keeping calories low on the down day activates SIRT1, which turns off the gene PPAR-gamma that is required for fat storage. This means that the Alternate-Day Diet preserves your muscle and you lose mostly fat, and the more SIRT1 is stimulated by keeping down-day calories low, the greater the effect.

This effect was demonstrated in the one-meal-a-day study conducted by Mattson and associates that we discussed on page 34. The people in this study who ate only one meal a day lost 4.6 pounds of fat but only 3.1 pounds of body weight. This means they *gained* 1.5 pounds of muscle even though they did not alter their physical activity. This is a remarkable result, because normally there would be loss of muscle with any degree of weight loss, and the reduction in body fat by 4.6 pounds is important because, as we have seen, it is the amount of body fat (or lack thereof) that determines health and longevity.

Q. *Does the Alternate-Day Diet cause ketosis?*

A. In the asthma-diet study, where subjects were consuming less than 20 percent of their daily required calories, they all showed an increase in ketone levels on the down day. Our clinical testing has indicated that if your intake is below 25 percent on the down day there is an increase in urine ketone level. Higher levels of ketones, which are sometimes seen in people whose calories come mainly from fat and protein (i.e., the Atkins Diet), are thought to help suppress appetite and improve stress resistance in the central nervous system. However, if your down day intake is 30 to 35 percent, most people following the Alternate-Day Diet don't show ketones in the urine.

Q. *Isn't the Alternate-Day Diet a kind of yo-yo dieting, and isn't that unhealthy?*

A. First of all, this diet has nothing at all to do with yo-yo dieting—or weight cycling, as it is called by researchers. "Yo-yo dieting" refers to the repeated loss and regaining of weight over a period of years. The Alternate-Day Diet restricts calories on alternate days in order to achieve permanent weight loss and improved health.

That said, however, it is not clear that the repeated loss and regaining of weight is necessarily harmful to health or if it is more harmful than remaining overweight. Although no one would encourage anyone to purposefully engage in yo-yo dieting, would it be better for people who have lost and gained weight over time to just give up and remain overweight?

Studies of weight cyclers have generally failed to show that they have a higher likelihood of dying or incidence of disease. One study found a lower effectiveness of natural killer cells (monocytes), which defend against viruses and cancer, in women who weight cycled, and the authors speculated that they might, therefore, be less healthy. However, other factors might have been operating; in calorie-restricted animals, the number of lymphocytes declines by one-third but are more effective than normal lymphocytes and the animals show better, not worse health. In healthy, middle-aged individuals, a history of weight cycling does not seem to increase the risk of long-term weight gain in men; however, this relation needs to be studied further in women.

At the moment, there is no definitive answer to the question of whether weight cycling is unhealthy in any way, while the evidence that being overweight causes poorer health is indisputable. It seems highly doubtful, therefore, that overweight people would be better off if they were told they could never be thin and it was hopeless for them to try. As stated by one researcher, "Without more compelling evidence of the risks of weight cycling, warnings overriding safe, effective weight-loss treatments for the obese are unwarranted."

Finally, there is the question of whether weight cycling makes long-term weight gain more likely. Studies do not indicate that weight gain or fat gain is more likely with weight cycling, nor is there evidence that it gets harder to lose weight with subsequent cycles. In all probability, regaining weight is the consequence of allowing ourselves to eat in an unrestrained and nutritionally undesirable way.

Q. *Could the Alternate-Day Diet lead to anorexia or another eating disorder?*

A. There have been comments that this diet could cause anorexia, but to date there has been no indication of any relationship between anorexia and the Alternate-Day Diet. I am not aware of anyone who has gone on this diet and subsequently become predisposed to this kind of problem, although there are always people who might abuse the Alternate-Day Diet—or any diet for that matter. In fact, anorexics would not be able to eat a normal amount of food on the up days. And bulimia, to my knowledge, has not been aggravated by the diet.

In 1992, the National Institutes of Health stated, "It is known that the onset of binge behavior occurs only after the experience of dieting." It also appears that the incidence of eating disorders is on the rise. According to an article in the February 1, 2007, issue of the *Journal of Biological Psychiatry*, 0.6 percent of the population has anorexia, 1 percent has bulimia, and 2.8 percent has a binge-eating disorder. These disorders are about twice as common among women as men and also correlate with a high incidence of other psychiatric problems: 94 percent of bulimics, 56 percent of anorexics, and 79 percent of binge eaters have another psychiatric diagnosis. One-half have major depression and one-third are substance abusers. Therefore, if you are experiencing emotional problems and think you might have an eating disorder, you should seek professional help before starting any diet program.

Q. If I eat every other day, won't I develop a vitamin deficiency?

A. No. Vitamin deficiency simply doesn't happen in just twenty-four hours. As long as you eat sensibly, and supplement as necessary, you won't have a problem. (You have a much higher chance of being vitamin deficient on a diet of fast food than on the Alternate-Day Diet.)

Q. Should I start on an up day or a down day?

A. If you're eating normally before you start the diet, technically speaking you'll have to start on a down day, although you can certainly choose to decide that you're starting on a normal eating day. One way or another, it doesn't really matter.

Q. How soon will I experience the positive effects of the Alternate-Day Diet?

A. Both the health effects and weight loss will be felt within the first three days, as they were for the people in our Asthma Study.

Q. How low should I go on the down day?

A. To maximize the response that lowers oxidative stress and inflammation, eating nothing every other day would probably be most effective. Except, of course, that no one can do it!

I originally conceived of the Alternate-Day Diet as eating 20 percent of normal on the down day because I estimated that this amount would be tolerable in terms of hunger control while simultaneously activating the calorie-restriction mechanism. It's proved to be acceptable to a large percentage of motivated dieters. Some individuals, however, find 20 percent to be too low and prefer 30 to 35 percent and have seen both weight loss and good health results at that level. I myself generally adhere to a 50 percent down-day level alternating with roughly 100 percent up days interspersed with days of 25 to 35 percent.

The effectiveness of any diet is completely contingent on the ability of the dieter to comply over time. Therefore, you need to determine the level you can tolerate for the long term.

Q. *I've heard that the most successful dieters are those who eat a good breakfast. Is that true, and how can I eat a good breakfast on my down days?*

A. There are numerous studies purporting to show better cognitive function and decreased tendency to overeat in people who eat breakfast. Records from the National Weight Control Registry, which tracks successful dieters, indicate that 78 percent of these people eat breakfast. The implied reasons are that skipping breakfast will just set you up to eat more when you finally get so hungry that you gorge, and also that eating breakfast jump-starts your metabolism to burn more calories. There is, however, no good scientific basis for either of these claims. Assumedly all those successful dieters became overweight by eating (at least) three meals a day. If you want to eat a good breakfast on your up days, please do!

Q. *What's the difference between having a shake and eating a five-hundred-calorie lunch, as some other diets recommend?*

A. Either one will work. The midday lunch is based on the notion that it helps you to reduce hunger and stay alert. However, most people like to have some calories in the morning and a small amount throughout the day, using either the shake or very low-calorie foods.

Q. *Don't you need to eat frequently to rev up your metabolism so that you burn more calories in order to lose weight?*

A. The answer to that question is a definitive no. This is one of the common myths about metabolism, but without any basis in physiology. While it is true that the process of digestion does expend some energy and, therefore, increases your metabolic rate, in order to have a net negative-calorie effect (and thus lose weight), the food you were eating would have to have fewer calories than the calories burned in digesting it. This might apply if you were eating sawdust, which is indigestible and would require some energy expenditure to push through the GI tract, but it would certainly not apply to eating any normal food. All normal food has more calories than what your body requires to digest it—that's why it's called *food*.

Q. *What do I do if I blow it on a down day?*

A. First off, realize that you have *begun*! You have made a conscious decision to follow the Alternate-Day Diet, and you are doing your best (which is all any of us can do). Second, no one can do this or any diet perfectly. Life gets in the way. Third, you can start over tomorrow. You will have some great down days and others when you will blow it. When you do, you have two choices: turn the down day into an up day or make the down day an in-between day. The worst thing to do is to succumb to all-or-nothing thinking that you may as well pig out since you've already blown it.

Q. *What happens if I miss a down day?*

A. SIRT1 is turned on by the low-calorie intake of the down day, remains active for more than twenty-four hours after the end of that day, and is probably present in decreasing concentration for several more days. The repetition of the down days increases SIRT1 protein levels to a maximum after approximately three weeks. Therefore, if you miss a down day after following the diet for some time you would experience a decline in SIRT1 protein levels but still have much of the desirable anti-inflammatory activity. If, on the other hand, you had only done one or two down days, you would not have achieved maximum stimulation of the SIRT1 response and would lose those benefits more quickly. If you stop the diet completely, it appears to take twenty-one days to lose most of the beneficial effects.

Q. *I don't want to do down days on the weekend. Can I do them on Monday, Wednesday, and Friday?*

A. Many people find it easiest to do Monday, Wednesday, and Friday down days and make either or both Saturday and Sunday up days. This works well and clearly maintains activation of the anti-inflammatory process. However, most people eat more on weekends, probably because they are not distracted by work and engage in more social activity. So, if you are trying to lose weight on the Alternate-Day Diet, you should exercise caution and keep an up-to-the-minute food log to remain conscious of what you are eating. As soon as you eat something, write it down.

Another strategy would be to make Sunday an "in-between" day, meaning that you still restrict to some extent but eat more than you would on a regular down day. Some alternate-day dieters have found that this works for them while others have found that calculating in-between day calories just adds to their stress and, therefore, becomes counterproductive. Again, as I've said before, it's a matter of knowing yourself and what works for you.

Q. *How does the Alternate-Day Diet compare to the 5/2 diet?*

A. The 5/2 diet is simply restricting calories two days a week rather than every other day. This may be easier for some people to do, and there is evidence that it would result in better health than doing nothing at all. Restricting calories even one day a month has been shown to improve health. But the Alternate-Day Diet provides the best results.

Q. *Can I do two down days in a row?*

A. You can, but it's very unpleasant, and you'll also be slowing your metabolic rate, which will counteract the benefits of the alternate-day pattern.

Q. *How much should I eat on the up day?*

A. To answer that question, it is important to understand the psychology of the Alternate-Day Diet, the point of which is to reduce stress and diet fatigue and increase freedom from the anxiety of restricting every day so that you are more likely to adhere to the diet over time.

Oddly, based on the Calorie Calculator (page 76), some dieters seem to believe that there is a number of calories they are *required* to eat on the up days. However, the sole purpose of using the Calorie Calculator is to estimate the number of calories to eat on your down days. You absolutely *do not* have to consume all the calories estimated for your up days. *There is no specific calorie requirement for the up day.*

The most important principle of the Alternate-Day Diet is to keep your down-day calories as low as practical while maintaining the up-day, down-day pattern over the long term.

Q. *What about carbs?*

A. This diet is strictly about calories, but many people find that minimizing "white foods," on both the up and down days, but especially on the up days, helps them lose weight. Since the down days are all about consuming low-calorie foods, this would naturally preclude sugary or starchy carbs. It's the calorie restriction that activates SIRT1—no matter where those calories come from. For more information on carbs and this diet, check out lowcarbfriends.com/bbs/juddd.

Q. *What about going "low carb" on the up day?*

A. We have covered the principles of good nutrition in Chapter 7, which you should keep in mind if you intend to follow the Alternate-Day Diet indefinitely. The answer to this question centers on understanding that if you are overweight, you are *always* going to have to control your eating. The only logical long-term solution—given the huge potential benefits—appears to be the practice of restraint every other day.

Following a plan of the traditional Atkins type, which includes large quantities of saturated fat, is not recommended. If you follow a plan with healthier sources of protein, such as chicken, fish, and low-fat dairy, you may find it more satiating. The bottom line is that if you are going to benefit from the modern science of nutrition, it is necessary to consume whole grains and non-starchy vegetables—that is, healthy carbohydrates—in sufficient quantities.

Some people have found it easier during the active weight-loss phase to follow a low-glycemic, high (healthy) protein diet on the up day, and then shift to a more vegetable-based diet once they reach their goal weight.

Q. Do I need to exercise?

A. Exercise is definitely essential for good health, but exercise alone will not cause significant weight loss. It is necessary to keep your down-day calorie intake to no more than 25 percent of normal to get the maximum benefit of the diet. This is important because many people use exercise as a handy excuse to eat more.

Thirty minutes of aerobic exercise daily and resistance training three times a week is a program most people are able to maintain. Those who do significantly more aerobic exercise can increase their down-day intake, but doing that is a slippery slope, because most people underestimate the number of calories they are consuming.

Q. How do I fit this plan into my family's lifestyle?

A. You can cook for your family in advance on your up days and refrigerate or freeze what you've cooked until needed. To avoid succumbing to hunger on your down days, try going for a walk while your family is eating, or join them at the table with a large bowl of greens dressed with vinegar and a teaspoonful of oil.

Q. *Will I gain weight if I go off the diet?*

A. Most people who lose weight on any diet regain it within a year or two. The Alternate-Day Diet appears to have a lower level of recidivism; however, the fact is that 90 percent of the population will gain weight over time in our cheap and available food environment. People who are successful with the Alternate-Day Diet make it a lifestyle, and if life prevents them from being consistent for some period of time, it's easy to restart.

Q. *How much is this diet going to cost me?*

A. Many diets require the purchase of specific, potentially expensive foods. This diet does not. The only additional cost would be the shakes I recommend for the first two weeks of the diet, but even those cost less than the food you would normally be buying to eat on your down days.

Acknowledgments

We would like to extend our thanks to the following people, without whom this book would not have been possible:

Sujit John, MS, of Stanford University Department of Statistics, for his outstanding statistical analysis of study data, his unstinting effort in assisting in research, and his many insights and friendship.

Mark Mattson, head of Neurosciences Laboratory at the National Institute on Aging, National Institutes of Health, for inspiring us through his contributions to basic science to undertake research on alternate-day calorie restriction, and his participation in and enormous contribution to our asthma/diet study.

Warren Summer, MD, section chief of Pulmonary/Critical Care Medicine at Louisiana State University Health Sciences Center, for assisting in design of the asthma/diet study and contributing his vast experience and help in managing the subjects with asthma, and for helping to write the article. Konrad Howitz at BIOMOL also assisted in the study design.

Our other NIH colleagues who assisted in assays and analysis of the results for the asthma/diet study, notably Roy Cutler, Bronwen Martin, Dong Hoon Hyun, and Vishwa Dixit. Rafael de Cabo, for his advice and assistance with essays.

The many scientists who have contributed to the ever-growing body of knowledge in the study of calorie restriction, including Clive McCay, Roy Walford, Edward Masoro, Don Ingram, Richard Weindruch, John Holloczy, and Luigi Fontana, and molecular biologists, including Leonard Guarente of MIT and David Sinclair of Harvard, who are adding almost daily to the understanding on a cellular level of the causes of aging.

Eric Ravussin, PhD, of the Pennington Biomedical Research Institute, and Marc Hellerstein, MD, of the University of California, for their very important contributions, consultation, and advice.

Susan Crawford, for her excellent transcription.

Mary Johnson; and daughters, Sarah, Dinah, and Genevieve (and Joey and Leo).

Dana Johnson, Joan Hailey, Cindy Klibert, and Heidi Pichon, for their assistance with the asthma/diet study and to the subjects who volunteered for the study.

Dick and Esther Paul, for their enthusiasm, encouragement, advice, and friendship.

Judy Kern, for reworking the manuscript, and Jeanette Egan, for providing the original recipes.

And John Duff, our publisher, without whom the book would not exist and who has provided so much to the final product.

Sources

Aksungar, F. B., Topkaya, A. E., and Akyildiz, M. Interleukin-6, C-reactive protein and biochemical parameters during prolonged intermittent fasting. *Ann. Nutr. Metab.* 2007; 51(1):88–95. PMID: 17374948.

Albu, J., and Reed, G. Weight cycling: more questions than answers. *Endocr. Pract.* 1995 Sep.–Oct.; 1(5):346–52. PMID: 15251582.

Anderson, J. W., Conley, S. B., and Nicholas, A. S. One-hundred-pound weight losses with an intensive behavioral program: changes in risk factors in 118 patients with long-term follow-up. *Am. J. Clin. Nutr.* 2007 Aug.; 86(2):301–7. PMID: 17684198.

Anson, R. M., Guo, Z., de Cabo, R., Iyun, T., Rios, M., Hagepanos, A., Ingram, D. K., Lane, M. A., and Mattson, M. P. Intermittent fasting dissociates beneficial effects of dietary restriction on glucose metabolism and neuronal resistance to injury from calorie intake. *Proc. Natl. Acad. Sci. U S A.* 2003 May 13; 100(10):6216–20. PMID: 12724520.

Armstrong, L. E. Caffeine, body fluid-electrolyte balance, and exercise performance. *Int. J. Sport Nutr. Exerc. Metab.* 2002 Jun.; 12(2): 189–206. PMID: 12187618.

Baur, J. A., Pearson, K. J., Price, N. L., Jamieson, H. A., Lerin, C.,

Kalra, A., Prabhu, V. V., Allard, J. S., Lopez-Lluch, G., Lewis, K., Pistell, P. J., Poosala, S., Becker, K. G., Boss, O., Gwinn, D., Wang, M., Ramaswamy, S., Fishbein, K. W., Spencer, R. G., Lakatta, E. G., Le Couteur, D., Shaw, R. J., Navas, P., Puigserver, P., Ingram, D. K., de Cabo, R., and Sinclair, D. A. Resveratrol improves health and survival of mice on a high-calorie diet. *Nature.* 2006 Nov. 16; 444(7117):337–42. PMID: 17086191.

Beatty, W. W., Clouse, B. A., and Bierley, R. A. Effects of long-term restricted feeding on radial maze performance by aged rats. *Neurobiol. Aging.* 1987 Jul.–Aug.; 8(4):325–7. PMID: 3627348.

Bjelakovic, G., Nikolova, D., Gluud, L. L., Simonetti, R. G., and Gluud, C. Mortality in randomized trials of antioxidant supplements for primary and secondary prevention: systematic review and meta-analysis. *JAMA.* 2007 Feb. 28; 297(8):842–57. PMID: 17327526.

Blackburn, G. L., and Rothacker, D. Ten-year self-management of weight using a meal replacement diet plan: comparison with matched controls. *Obes. Res.* 2003; 11:A103.

Boston Collaborative Drug Surveillance Group. Regular aspirin intake and acute myocardial infarction. *Br. Med. J.* 1974; 1:440–3. PMID: 4816857.

Bruce-Keller, A. J., Umberger, G., McFall, R., and Mattson, M. P. Food restriction reduces brain damage and improves behavioral outcome following excitotoxic and metabolic insults. *Ann. Neurol.* 1999 Jan.; 45(1):8–15. PMID: 9894871.

Cawthon, R. M., Smith, K. R., O'Brien, E., Sivatchenko, A., and Kerber, R. A. Association between telomere length in blood and mortality in people aged 60 years or older. *Lancet.* 2003 Feb. 1; 361(9355): 393–5. PMID: 12573379.

Chan, J. L., Mietus, J. E., Raciti, P. M., Goldberger, A. L., and Mantzoros, C. S. Short-term fasting-induced autonomic activation and changes in catecholamine levels are not mediated by changes in leptin levels in healthy humans. *Clin. Endocrinol.* (Oxf.). 2007 Jan.; 66(1):49–57. PMID: 17201801.

Cutler D. M., Glaeser, E. L., and Shapiro, J. M. Why have Americans become more obese? *J. Econ. Perspect.* 2003; 17:93–118.

Descamps, O., Riondel, J., Ducros, V., and Roussel, A. M. Mitochondrial production of reactive oxygen species and incidence of age-associated lymphoma in OF1 mice: effect of alternate-day fasting. *Mech. Ageing Dev.* 2005 Nov.; 126(11):1185–91. PMID: 16126250.

Elias, M. F., Elias, P. K., Sullivan, L. M., Wolf, P. A., and D'Agostino, R. B. Lower cognitive function in the presence of obesity and hypertension: the Framingham heart study. *Int. J. Obes. Relat. Metab. Disord.* 2003 Feb.; 27(2):260–8. PMID: 12587008.

Flegal, K. M., Graubard, B. I., Williamson, D. F., and Gail, M. H. Excess deaths associated with underweight, overweight, and obesity. *JAMA.* 2005 Apr. 20; 293(15):1861–7. PMID: 15840860.

Heilbronn, L. K, Smith, S. R., Martin, C. K., Anton, S. D., and Ravussin, E. Alternate-day fasting in nonobese subjects: effects on body weight, body composition, and energy metabolism. *Am. J. Clin. Nutr.* 2005 Jan.; 81(1):69–73. PMID: 15640462.

Heitmann, B. L., Erikson, H., Ellsinger, B. M., Mikkelsen, K. L., and Larsson, B. Mortality associated with body fat, fat-free mass and body mass index among 60-year-old Swedish men—a 22-year follow-up. The study of men born in 1913. *Int. J. Obes. Relat. Metab. Disord.* 2000 Jan.; 24(1):33–7. PMID: 10702748.

Hsieh, E. A., Chai, C. M., and Hellerstein, M. K. Effects of caloric restriction on cell proliferation in several tissues in mice: role of intermittent feeding. *Am. J. Physiol. Endocrinol. Metab.* 2005 May; 288(5):E965–72. PMID: 15613681.

Hung, H. C., Joshipura, K. J., Jiang, R., Hu, F. B., Hunter, D., Smith-Warner, S. A., Colditz, G. A., Rosner, B., Spiegelman, D., and Willett, W. C. Fruit and vegetable intake and risk of major chronic disease. *J. Natl. Cancer Inst.* 2004 Nov. 3; 96(21):1577–84. PMID: 15523086.

Johnson, J. B., Laub, D. R., and John, S. The effect on health of alternate day calorie restriction: eating less and more than needed on alternate days prolongs life. *Med. Hypotheses.* 2006; 67(2):209–11.

Johnson, J. B., Summer, W., Cutler, R. G., Martin, B., Hyun, D. H., Dixit, V. D., Pearson, M., Nassar, M., Telljohann, R., Maudsley, S., Carlson, O., John, S., Laub, D. R., and Mattson, M. P. Alternate day calorie restriction improves clinical findings and reduces markers of oxidative stress and inflammation in overweight adults with moderate asthma. *Free Rad. Biol. Med.* 2007 Mar. 1; 42(5):665–74. PMID: 17291990.

Kaeberlein, M., McVey, M., and Guarente, L. The SIR2/3/4 complex and SIR2 alone promote longevity in Saccharomyces cerevisiae by two different mechanisms. *Genes. Dev.* 1999 Oct. 1; 13(19):2570–80. PMID: 10521401.

Kim, D., Nguyen, M. D., Dobbin, M. M., Fischer, A., Sananbenesi, F., Rodgers, J. T., Delalle, I., Baur, J. A., Sui, G., Armour, S. M., Puigserver, P., Sinclair, D. A., and Tsai, L. H. SIRT1 deacetylase protects against neurodegeneration in models for Alzheimer's disease and amyotrophic lateral sclerosis. *EMBO J.* 2007 Jul. 11; 26(13):3169–79. PMID: 17581637.

Lagouge, M., Argmann, C., Gerhart-Hines, Z., Meziane, H., Lerin, C., Daussin, F., Messadeq, N., Milne, J., Lambert, P., Elliott, P., Geny, B., Laakso, M., Puigserver, P., and Auwerx, J. Resveratrol improves mitochondrial function and protects against metabolic disease by activating SIRT1 and PGC-1alpha. *Cell.* 2006 Dec. 15; 127(6):1109–22. PMID: 17112576.

Lichtman, S. W., Pisarska, K., Berman, E. R., Pestone, M., Dowling, H., Offenbacher, E., Weisel, H., Heshka, S., Matthews, D. E., and Heymsfield, S. B. Discrepancy between self-reported and actual caloric intake and exercise in obese subjects. *N. Engl. J. Med.* 1992 Dec. 31; 327(27):1893–8. PMID: 1454084.

Mair, W., Goymer, P., Pletcher, S. D., and Partridge, L. Demography of dietary restriction and death in Drosophila. *Science.* 2003 Sep. 19; 301(5640):1731–3. PMID: 14500985.

McCay, C. M., Crowell, M. F., Maynard, L. A. The effect of retarded growth upon the length of life and upon ultimate size. *J. Nutr.* 1935; 10:63–79.

Molarius, A., Seidell, J. C., Sans, S., Tuomilehto, J., and Kuulasmaa, K. Educational level, relative body weight, and changes in their association over 10 years: an international perspective from the WHO

MONICA Project. *Am. J. Public Health.* 2000 Aug.; 90(8):1260–8. PMID: 10937007.

Mukamal, K. J., Conigrave, K. M., Mittleman, M. A., Camargo, C. A., Jr., Stampfer, M. J., Willett, W. C., and Rimm, E. B. Roles of drinking pattern and type of alcohol consumed in coronary heart disease in men. *N. Engl. J. Med.* 2003 Jan. 9; 348(2):109–18. PMID: 12519921.

Philipson, T., Dai, C., Helmchen, L., and Variyam, J. The economics of obesity: a report on the workshop held at USDA's Economic Research Service. Economic Research Service, USDA E-FAN No. 04004, May 2004 (ers.usda.gov/media/328677/efan04004fm_1_.pdf).

Philipson, T. J., and Posner, R. A. The long-run growth in obesity as a function of technological change. *Perspect Biol. Med.* 2003 Summer; 46(3 Suppl.):S87–107. PMID: 14563077.

Picard, F., Kurtev, M., Chung, N., Topark-Ngarm, A., Senawong, T., Machado De Oliveira, R., Leid, M., McBurney, M. W., and Guarente, L. Sirt1 promotes fat mobilization in white adipocytes by repressing PPAR-gamma. *Nature.* 2004 Jun. 17; 429(6993):771–6. PMID: 15175761.

Rodgers, J. T., Lerin, C., Haas, W., Gygi, S. P., Spiegelman, B. M., and Puigserver, P. Nutrient control of glucose homeostasis through a complex of PGC-1alpha and SIRT1. *Nature.* 2005 Mar. 3; 434 (7029):113–8. PMID: 15744310.

Roza, A. M., and Shizgal, H. M. The Harris Benedict equation reevaluated: resting energy requirements and the body cell mass. *Am. J. Clin. Nutr.* 1984 Jul.; 40(1):168–82. PMID: 6741850.

Shishehbor, M. H., Aviles, R. J., Brennan, M. L., Fu, X., Goormastic, M., Pearce, G. L., Gokce, N., Keaney, J. F. Jr., Penn, M. S., Sprecher, D. L., Vita, J. A., and Hazen, S. L. Association of nitrotyrosine levels with cardiovascular disease and modulation by statin therapy. *JAMA.* 2003 Apr. 2; 289(13):1675–80. PMID: 12672736.

Stewart, J., Mitchell, J., and Kalant, N. The effects of life-long food restriction on spatial memory in young and aged Fischer 344 rats measured in the eight-arm radial and the Morris water mazes. *Neurobiol. Aging.* 1989 Nov.–Dec.; 10(6):669–75. PMID: 2628778.

Stote, K. S., Baer, D. J., Spears, K., Paul, D. R., Harris, G. K., Rumpler, W. V., Strycula, P., Najjar, S. S., Ferrucci, L., Ingram, D. K., Longo, D. L., and Mattson, M.P. A controlled trial of reduced meal frequency without caloric restriction in healthy, normal-weight, middle-aged adults. *Am. J. Clin. Nutr.* 2007 Apr.; 85(4):981–8. PMID: 17413096.

Thomas, E. J., Abrams, K. S., and Johnson, J. B. Self-monitoring and the reciprocal inhibition in the modification of multiple tics of Gilles de la Tourette's syndrome. *J. Behav. Ther. Exp. Psychiatry.* 1971; 2: 159–171 (http://hdl.handle.net/2027.42/33572).

Vainio, H., and Bianchini, F. *IARC Handbooks of Cancer Prevention, vol. 6: Weight Control and Physical Activity.* Lyon, France: IARC Press, 2002.

Vallejo, E. A. La dieta de hambre a dias alternos en la alimentacion de los viejos. *Rev. Clin. Esp.* 1956; 63:25–7.

Valtin, H. "Drink at least eight glasses of water a day." Really? Is there scientific evidence for "8 x 8"? *Am. J. Physiol. Regul. Integr. Comp. Physiol.* 2002 Nov.; 283(5):R993–1004. PMID: 12376390.

Wang, Y., Monteiro, C., and Popkin, B. M. Trends of obesity and underweight in older children and adolescents in the United States, Brazil, China, and Russia. *Am. J. Clin. Nutr.* 2002 Jun.; 75(6):971–7. PMID: 12036801.

Zeller, J. L., Burke, A. E., and Glass, R. M. JAMA patient page. Acute appendicitis in children. *JAMA.* 2007 Jul. 25; 298(4):482. PMID: 17652303.

Index

About the Authors

James B. Johnson, MD, an instructor in plastic surgery at Louisiana State University School of Medicine, retired after more than twenty years in private practice to pursue his longtime interest in alternate-day calorie restriction. He has published numerous articles in peer-reviewed journals, including *Medical Hypotheses* and *Free Radical Biology & Medicine*. His work has also been featured in the popular press, including the *Independent* (London) and *Woman's World*. He lives in Metairie, Louisiana.

Donald R. Laub Sr , MD, is an adjunct clinical associate professor of surgery at Stanford University and a founder of Interplast, the first humanitarian organization to provide free reconstructive surgery for children with clefts, disabling burns, and hand injuries. The author of more than one hundred scientific papers, he has received numerous humanitarian and service awards.

Visit Dr. Johnson's website at alternatedaydiet.com.